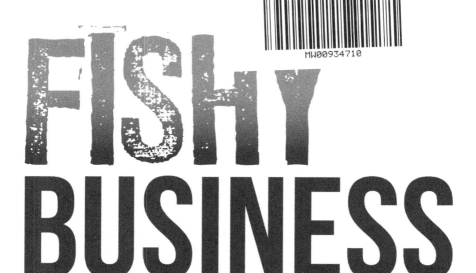

FISHY
BUSINESS

WHY FISH OILS
CAN DO MORE HARM
THAN GOOD

YOURI KRUSE

Foreword **RAYMOND PEAT, PHD**   Introduction **PETR GRÚZ, PHD**

On a personal note, I know that both DHA and EPA could have vital functions in the human body, such as the maturation of neurons and some brain functions. Usually, the case is made, especially with DHA, for peroxisome diseases like Zellweger's disease. But some studies show that even these conditions are not always improved by DHA and are not seen as causally linked[12]. My opinion is that in the average diet, intake of these fats has already been excessive if we can reduce omega-6. Any experimentation on the reader's part is their responsibility.

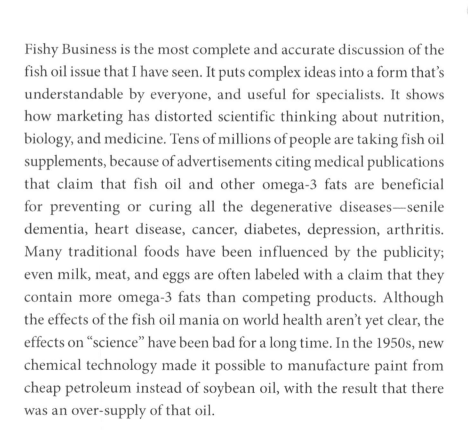

FOREWORD

Raymond Peat, PhD

Fishy Business is the most complete and accurate discussion of the fish oil issue that I have seen. It puts complex ideas into a form that's understandable by everyone, and useful for specialists. It shows how marketing has distorted scientific thinking about nutrition, biology, and medicine. Tens of millions of people are taking fish oil supplements, because of advertisements citing medical publications that claim that fish oil and other omega-3 fats are beneficial for preventing or curing all the degenerative diseases—senile dementia, heart disease, cancer, diabetes, depression, arthritis. Many traditional foods have been influenced by the publicity; even milk, meat, and eggs are often labeled with a claim that they contain more omega-3 fats than competing products. Although the effects of the fish oil mania on world health aren't yet clear, the effects on "science" have been bad for a long time. In the 1950s, new chemical technology made it possible to manufacture paint from cheap petroleum instead of soybean oil, with the result that there was an over-supply of that oil.

Two articles published in 1929 and 1930 by George and Mildred Burr, that had claimed that a trace amount of linoleic or linolenic acid was an essential nutrient for animals, were seen as an opportunity for marketing the liquid vegetable oils.

Although it was difficult, if not impossible, to create a deficiency disease by eliminating those oils, any suggestion that these agricultural by-product oils had nutritional value was enough to create huge advertising campaigns to sell them for human consumption. Other research was identified that the industry used to promote the use of massive amounts of these oils: The idea that solid animal fats cause heart disease was twisted into the idea that liquid vegetables oils would protect against heart disease. By the 1970s, this jumble of pseudo-scientific advertising claims was being challenged by the growing evidence that an excess of polyunsaturated fats—"essential fatty acids"—in the diet causes cancer, heart disease, and many other problems. As it was becoming impossible to deny the toxicity of the "essential" linoleic acid, it happened that the fishing industry had been experiencing problems in disposing of large amounts of fish oil, and a combination of advertising and subsidized research was able to sell the idea that the toxicity of the essential fatty acids was just a matter of balance, which could be overcome by ingesting fish oils. While advertising was changing the way people were advised to eat, it was also changing the way researchers thought about the composition of the human body, and the way it changes with age. The fact that the developing fetus makes its own polyunsaturated fats from glucose is distorted, interpreting the presence of these natural brain lipids as evidence of a deficiency of essential fatty acids, justifying neonatal, or even prenatal, supplementation of the omega-3 fats, especially DHA and EPA, the characteristic fats of fish oil. Ideas about other stages of life have been similarly distorted. I hope Fishy Business will give people the knowledge and the courage to resist the pressures to give "essential fatty acid" supplements to their families, even when they are prescribed by doctors. Informed patients can become the most effective method of medical education.

Raymond Peat, PhD

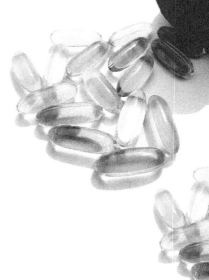

INTRODUCTION

Petr Grúz, PhD
My lifelong experience with oils and ω-3

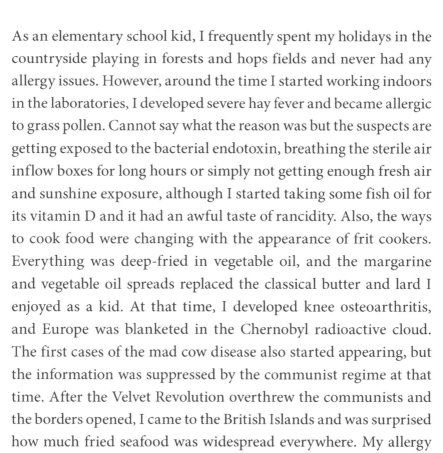

As an elementary school kid, I frequently spent my holidays in the countryside playing in forests and hops fields and never had any allergy issues. However, around the time I started working indoors in the laboratories, I developed severe hay fever and became allergic to grass pollen. Cannot say what the reason was but the suspects are getting exposed to the bacterial endotoxin, breathing the sterile air inflow boxes for long hours or simply not getting enough fresh air and sunshine exposure, although I started taking some fish oil for its vitamin D and it had an awful taste of rancidity. Also, the ways to cook food were changing with the appearance of frit cookers. Everything was deep-fried in vegetable oil, and the margarine and vegetable oil spreads replaced the classical butter and lard I enjoyed as a kid. At that time, I developed knee osteoarthritis, and Europe was blanketed in the Chernobyl radioactive cloud. The first cases of the mad cow disease also started appearing, but the information was suppressed by the communist regime at that time. After the Velvet Revolution overthrew the communists and the borders opened, I came to the British Islands and was surprised how much fried seafood was widespread everywhere. My allergy worsened, and I even started getting sort of asthmatic attacks from the flowering grass fields in Europe, so it was a big relief when I moved to the damp Japan, where the grass is relatively scarce as the country is mostly covered with volcanic rocks. The ordinary Japanese food is also heavily fried, but there is a choice of healthier raw alternatives such as sushi or other classical rice and soy-based dishes. However, I continued my old eating habits thriving on margarine and eating the bento packed with fried items with some ω-3 rich fish occasionally. The allergy did not go away.

I never paid any attention to the fatty acids until one day when I heard the hypothesis that the trans fats in margarine and shortening were responsible for the explosive rise in allergies in the modern world. That was a big motivation to look into this issue, and I asked the key question – if trans fats are bad, then what should we substitute for it? The surrounding people answered simply, healthy fats! Then I looked up what the healthy fats were on the Internet, and the answer coming from everywhere was – the fats rich in ω-3 fatty acids! Wow, that looked simple. I also read how ω-3 fatty acids fight cancer. Cancer was the disease which scared me pretty much as my mother died from it young, my father has been battling it, and even my great teacher in science was in its terminal stage. Moreover, I also remember attending a lecture of the president of the National Cancer Center in which he was sharing how young and how many of his employees were dying from different types of cancer. So I started experimenting with my health and at first picked up the Budwig Diet using flaxseed oil. But it did not help my allergy issues and I strangely started getting out of breath even when riding a small slope on my bicycle. Furthermore, at home, we substituted the refined flax seed oil rich in the ω-3 linolenic acid for the conventional ω-6 linoleic acid, rich cooking oils and shortening, what later turned out to be a fatal mistake. While ingesting this unstable oil oxidized at high cooking temperatures, I started having really bothering vision problems with the appearance of eye floaters, then my knee osteoarthritis worsened, and I tore the meniscus during a normal run and wasn't able to walk normally.

Again, I started seeking a solution and found that the inflammation in my knees could be stopped with fish oil, which contains the long-chain ω-3 fatty acids like DHA, which are more powerful immunomodulators than their precursors from the flaxseed oil. The Internet is heavily polluted with information about the health benefits of fish oil supplements containing the ω-3. I also added the borage oil rich in another anti-inflammatory ω-6 fatty acid GLA and threw some antioxidants like vitamin E and tomatoes for their lycopene into my supplement mix. My test of carotenoid antioxidant content in blood using the Pharmanex scanner came out excellent. My knee improved because I followed the advice to strengthen the muscle, holding it together and used the prolotherapy to avoid arthroscopic surgery. But I nearly died one day when I lost consciousness during a severe hypoglycemic episode and was found to have damaged leaky gut with multiple food intolerances as a consequence. Well, that was enough; something was not right here. After a couple of sleepless nights searching in the darkest places on the Internet, I found something interesting pointing towards the Ray Peat's site I have never been to before. It was written in the scientific language I was familiar with and suddenly, everything started making sense.

It was a thrill to start finding the scientific evidence in peer review journals showing e.g. how different species evolved their longevity by minimizing the utilization of the highly unstable building blocks composed of the ω-3 fatty acids, or how the mice deficient in the PUFAs, deemed to be essential, are resistant to cancer. It was even more fascinating when I started seeing the links to my professional work on mutagenesis and carcinogenesis. I suddenly saw the whole forest, which I couldn't previously see for the trees. Unfortunately, this topic was too difficult to discuss with most researchers in Japan, including my superiors, or they did not want to hear, except my former student, who had a deep interest in the nutrition and health sciences. As I badly needed to get back on track, I promptly adapted a new diet minimizing the exposure to all ω-6 and ω-3 PUFAs as much as practically possible and started seeing some amazing results. The energy came back, and I could easily ride my bicycle uphill, osteoarthritis went into remission, the spider veins on my ankles disappeared, and I did not catch any seasonal flu that year. I was in the best shape since coming to Japan. But from the scientific point of view, this is all just anecdotal evidence and could have been just a placebo effect. Although I found the theories put forward by Ray Peat quite appealing and being examined in some real-life situations such as at the Functional Performance Systems gym, this really should be verified by the Scientific method if not for anything else but the sake of humanity. To be able to rewrite the textbooks, a double-blind clinical trial or animal experiment is badly needed to obtain some solid evidence. Because this would cost a lot of time and money, no one is eager to put at stake their career to realize it now.

The Science

My efforts to apply for funding to realize the verification experiment, which would clearly demonstrate how essential and damaging or beneficial the essential fatty acids really are have been systematically suppressed by my superiors. Therefore, I resort to only using the tools allowed by my employer, which are the so-called "*in vitro*" bacterial mutagenicity tests, to gather evidence about potential human carcinogenicity. There has been some work done on the mutagenicity of the etheno-DNA adduct, forming lipid peroxidation products of the ω-3 fatty acids [I], which inspired me to test the mutagenicity of the related propano-DNA adduct forming compounds for the first time. This was also because the major propano-dG adduct represents a native substrate for the DNA polymerase κ, which I have been studying for a long time. This polymerase is an interesting enzyme since it seems to counteract the DNA damage from lipid peroxidation accumulating during the aging process. My results presented at several international conferences and published in the journal Mutation Research/ Genetic Toxicology and Environmental Mutagenesis [II] added to the growing amount of evidence that fish oil is not as healthy as generally thought. But the message is difficult to communicate to the regulatory authorities since the biochemists understand just the biochemistry, geneticists just the DNA mutations, and the nutritionists don't understand the biochemistry of mutagenesis at all. The implications of my findings for human carcinogenesis have been summarized at the 6th Asian Congress on Environmental Mutagens as follows [III] :

Endogenous lipid peroxide mediated DNA damage plays a key role in the aging process and can initiate cancer. Despite its high toxicity in bacteria, we have demonstrated the mutagenicity of major ω-3 fatty acid peroxidation products in the classical Ames test. 4-HHE is a neurotoxin derived from the docosahexaenoic acid (DHA), the most abundant ω-3 fatty acid in the human brain. It is clearly mutagenic in the mouse lymphoma assay and has been shown to form a cyclic $N2$-dG DNA adduct *in vitro*. Although the genotoxic risks from 4-HHE could be downplayed by recent work suggesting a hormetic response, some worrying data about the carcinogenic effects of long term exposure to the ω-3 fatty acids should not be ignored. This particularly includes the involvement of ω-3 PUFAs in prostate and breast tumorigenesis. A recent trend of balancing high ω-6 intake in modern diet with increased ω-3 consumption can prove quite dangerous if one considers the ω-3 PUFAs as initiators and ω-6 PUFAs as promoters of cancer. The role of ω-6 PUFAs in cancer promotion through the eicosanoid metabolism is widely acknowledged and demonstrated experimentally e.g. on the mouse skin cancer model. 4-HHE has been found at high levels in baby milk formula, spontaneously forms in the gastric and intestinal lumens after consuming fish meat as well as in human tissues. Other carcinogenic lipid peroxides such as crotonaldehyde are also formed by spontaneous oxidation of the ω-3 fatty acids. It is unlikely that DNA polymerase κ can undo all the genomic damage from lipid peroxidation since its competitor, the highly mutagenic TLS DNA polymerase ζ, is also activated in response to oxidized lipids.

Surviving In The Real World

Staying on an essential fatty acid semi-deficient diet is quite difficult in the nowadays world as all pre-made foods are laden with the seed oils, so one would have to prepare all food from scratch, and even then it may be difficult. E.g. the ruminant cattle fed its natural feed, which is grass, keeps special microbes in its second stomach, where these microorganisms biohydrogenate the plant PUFAs resulting in meat with relatively low PUFA content having some trans-fatty acids of microbial origin instead [IV]. But the common industrial meat is made by fattening the cattle with grains, and because the microbes would turn this unnatural food, due to its high starch content, into gasses, which would blow the cows up, the cattle are given antibiotics killing the microbes resulting in the seed-derived PUFAs going straight into the meat we then eat. Similarly, the fish raised on corn in farms like the salmon or tilapia incorporate the ω-6 arachidonic acid instead of the ω-3 DHA+EPA in the fish meat [V]. All bakeries are putting vegetable oils in their products to keep them soft and last longer. While studying the evolution of our nutrition, I arrived at the conclusion that humans have originally evolved as frugivores with a shift to some meat and animal fat-based diet as they moved to the north with seasonal root vegetables and nuts, but not the grains or beans. The tropical fruit is, in fact, rich in saturated fatty acids, and the ω-6 rich grains are the primary food for birds who have adaptations to properly digest them and deal with the unstable PUFAs in their membranes by e.g. decreasing the cysteine content of the mitochondrial energy-producing enzymes. The very powerful bird muscle needed for liftoff and flight, as well as the muscle of some top runner wild animals seems to take advantage of the arachidonic acid. In contrast to ω-3, the ω-6 arachidonic acid-derived eicosanoids are very powerful signaling molecules in the immune system acting during growth, reproduction and muscle regeneration, but backfire badly when in excess and out of the control especially in an aged organism. At least in humans, the most stable ω-9 mead acid seems to be the best fit for structural purposes since it is naturally present in the young, healthy tissues like the cartilage. Also, the fact that vertebrates cannot manufacture the ω-3 and ω-6 fatty acid in contrast to ω-9 is not just an evolutionary mistake.

Eventually, I found it quite difficult to stick to the PUFA avoidance diet long term, particularly at busy and stressful times like when the Fukushima nuclear reactors blew up or during the moving of our institute and adapting to living in new places. Thus, I went back to the catered food, which is primarily based on fried items, and new health problems started reappearing. But being more knowledgeable than ever before, I have developed personal strategies to keep the negative effect of the vegetable oil-laden food at bay. To offset the pro-inflammatory effects of the arachidonic acid, the key point is to not let it accumulate in the body by staying active and using the muscle, which consumes a lot of it. For the rest eating some wild fish, meat helps to balance the ω-6 with ω-3 but not using the fish oil, which lacks the protective furan fatty acids quenching the radicals [VI]. This is a big problem with the refined oils in general since the healthy oils like the sesame, or extra virgin olive oils contain specific natural inhibitors of the arachidonic acid metabolism. Since with the PUFA based diets excessive lipid peroxidation cannot be avoided, especially in an organism beyond its reproductive age, it is important to sustain the proper redox balance to eliminate the harmful products by natural detoxification mechanisms. This can be achieved by ensuring to get all the essential vitamins and co-factors with particular emphasis on the B-vitamin series. The biochemical evidence that the PUFAs considered to be essential do a lot of harm in the body is overwhelming, and I have summarized some of this in the book Molecular Basis of Nutrition and Aging [VII]. Some damage can be seen by naked eyes, particularly in the aged population, as the accumulation of oxidized ω-6 and ω-3 fatty acids e.g. at the age spots (lipofuscin), arterial plaques (oxidized cholesterol), in the eye retina (drusen) and felt as the non-pleasant smell of the elderly caused by 2-nonenal [VIII]. 2-nonenal is a cousin of 4-HNE known to be responsible for mutating the p53 tumor suppressor gene in human cancers, and both of them are derived from the seed oils in our diet. It remains to be assessed experimentally what would accumulate in these places if the dietary ω-6 and ω-3 PUFAs are avoided. There is some evidence that the ω-9 PUFAs can substitute for nearly all functions of the more unstable ω-6 and ω-3 PUFAs to sustain life [IX]. Of course, avoiding the polyunsaturated oils would not completely prevent the human aging, which runs on an (epi) genetic clock, that would be another story, but I believe it can make it graceful and painless.

The book Fishy Business is a rare piece of evidence gathering art that exposes the dark side of fortifying human nutrition with the highly unstable PUFAs from different angles. I hope the professional, as well as ordinary readers, will find it informative and like it. I think that reading the following chapters can help anyone to make a proper judgment about whether to consume the fish and similar oils without having to endure the trial and error journey like I did. I also hope this book will send a message to the regulatory authorities to finally re-evaluate the concentrated PUFAs added to our food chain for their long term safety.

Disclaimer

All the statements written in this section are my personal opinion and don't represent the official stance of my employer in any way. They are not intended to prevent, diagnose, or treat any disease.

REFERENCES

I. Maekawa M, Kawai K, Takahashi Y, Nakamura H, Watanabe T, Sawa R, Hachisuka K, Kasai H (2006) Identification of 4-Oxo-2-hexenal and Other Direct Mutagens Formed in Model Lipid Peroxidation Reactions as dGuo Adducts. *Chem Res Toxicol* 19: 130–138.

II. Grúz P, Shimizu M, Sugiyama K, Honma, M (2017) Mutagenicity of ω-3 fatty acid peroxidation products in the Ames test. *Mutat Res Toxicol Environ Mutagen* 819: 14–19.

III. Grúz P, Shimizu M, Yamada M, Sugiyama K, Honma, M (2019) Mechanisms of mutagenicity of ω-3 fatty acid peroxidation products. *The 6th Asian Congress on Environmental Mutagens*, Tokyo.

IV. Wang Y, Jacome-Sosa MM, Proctor SD (2012) The role of ruminant trans fat as a potential nutraceutical in the prevention of cardiovascular disease. *Food Res Int* 46: 460–468.

V. Weaver KL, Ivester P, Chilton JA, Wilson MD, Pandey P, Chilton FH (2008) The Content of Favorable and Unfavorable Polyunsaturated Fatty Acids Found in Commonly Eaten Fish. *J Am Diet Assoc* 108: 1178–1185.

VI. Spiteller G (2005) The relation of lipid peroxidation processes with atherogenesis: A new theory on atherogenesis. *Mol Nutr Food Res* 49: 999–1013.

VII. Grúz P (2016) Chapter 12 - Lipid Peroxidation, Diet, and the Genotoxicology of Aging. In Malavolta M, Mocchegiani E (eds.), *Molecular Basis of Nutrition and Aging* pp 155–176. Academic Press, San Diego.

VIII. Ishino K, Wakita C, Shibata T, Toyokuni S, Machida S, Matsuda S, Matsuda T, Uchida K (2010) Lipid Peroxidation Generates Body Odor Component *trans* -2-Nonenal Covalently Bound to Protein *in Vivo*. *J Biol Chem* 285: 15302–15313.

IX. Grúz P, Shimizu M (2010) Origins of age-related DNA damage and dietary strategies for its reduction. *Rejuvenation Res* 13: 285–287.

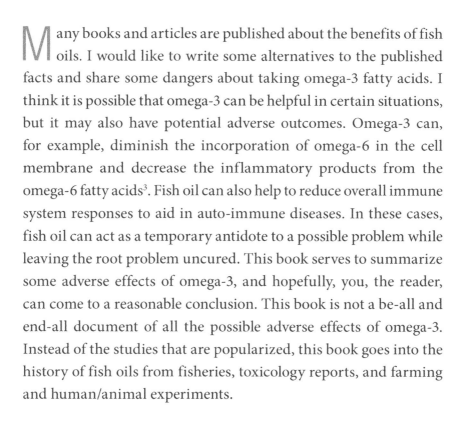

CHAPTER 1

Another Book About Fish Oil

M any books and articles are published about the benefits of fish oils. I would like to write some alternatives to the published facts and share some dangers about taking omega-3 fatty acids. I think it is possible that omega-3 can be helpful in certain situations, but it may also have potential adverse outcomes. Omega-3 can, for example, diminish the incorporation of omega-6 in the cell membrane and decrease the inflammatory products from the omega-6 fatty acids[3]. Fish oil can also help to reduce overall immune system responses to aid in auto-immune diseases. In these cases, fish oil can act as a temporary antidote to a possible problem while leaving the root problem uncured. This book serves to summarize some adverse effects of omega-3, and hopefully, you, the reader, can come to a reasonable conclusion. This book is not a be-all and end-all document of all the possible adverse effects of omega-3. Instead of the studies that are popularized, this book goes into the history of fish oils from fisheries, toxicology reports, and farming and human/animal experiments.

When one takes a historical perspective into account, a more reasonable view of fish oils can emerge. One of the most well-known facts about fish oil is its fragility. From a medical standpoint, fish oil was potentially so dangerous, that it was recommended only under stringent conditions.

"In connection with the above, it is evident the quality of medicinal fish oil used as a medicinal and prophylactic remedy should be rigidly controlled."[14]

FISHERIES RESEARCH BOARD OF CANADA Translation Series No. 2045, 'Effect of medicinal cod liver 'oil containing different amounts of aldehydes on the organism' (found here http://www.dfo-mpo.gc.ca/Library/13607.pdf). From the Fisheries and Oceans Canada

About Me

I am not a medical doctor nor a scientist. I am an independent researcher and a personal trainer. I have a degree in Sport and Health and have always been interested in science journals and books. My perception of the omega-3 fatty acids was positive as they protect against omega-6 inflammatory pathways. After reading Ray Peat's books and articles, I slowly changed my mind, and this book is my journey trying to figure out the nature, use, and health effects of fish oils. During this writing of this book, I found Peat's views are often echoed in academic circles regarding fish oil supplementation. I have accumulated many studies from the past that paint a different picture of the current view on fish oils. This book should not be used for any other purpose than for general information.

Health Supplement

This book summarizes my findings researching fish oil supplements. The research regarding fish oil involves positive, negative, and neutral effects and outcomes. The attention, however, lays most of the focus on positive studies. This book focuses on reasons why I don't take fish oil supplements as I think the possible adverse effects can outweigh the positive impact. Alternative tactics can instead gain these positive effects. In 2011, researchers at the University of Tohoku, Japan, showed that feeding fish oil to mice shortened their lifespan and increased inflammation[5]. The published study was met with an immediate editorial response arguing why the Tohoku study might not be correct[6]. The rebuttal on the Tokyo side ended with a letter which message is echoed in this book.

The author(s) wrote:

"we want to emphasize that a long-term intake of W-3 fatty acids (fish oil) may possibly damage health...It is not correct that w-3 fatty acids have only beneficial effects and it is important to know the risk. In fact, it has been previously reported that oxidative stress is increased by taking w-3 fatty acids..., and such inconvenient data should not be disregarded"[7]

Tsuduki T. Reply to Dr. Kang's letter entitled "Effect of ω-3 fatty acids on lifespan". Nutrition. 2011;27(6):731–732. doi:10.1016/j.nut.2011.03.001. Permission from Elsevier.

Fish Oil In The Media

When a 2015 New Zealand study found that most of the fish oil supplements showed a high rate of rancidity and that the levels of breakdown products were higher than recommended[8], the interesting part was not the limited publicity it received. The surprising part was the response from the fish oil industry that was published a year later. This study found that omega-3 oils in supplement form are not oxidized and safe[9]. The authors of the rebuttal study comprised of scientists who speak at symposiums sponsored by edible oils manufacturers, work for pharmaceutical companies and are advisors with the omega-3-center or (at the time of this writing) a center that is associated and aligned with the Global Organization for EPA and DHA (GOED). The rebuttal study stated no conflict of interest.

GOED Isn't That GOOD

Global Organization for EPA and DHA Omega-3s (GOED) is a non-profit organization that is funding studies regarding omega-3 and influences regulations for the omega-3 industry. GOED has about 200 members that are involved in the production and sales of, among other items, fish oil.

A short rundown of GOED activities includes

- Setting up ambassador networks with health professionals to "educate" consumers
- Funding of omega-3 studies (especially meta-analysis studies)
- Organizing events to promote omega-3 in the media

- Making recommendations for safety and standards for omega-3

GOED has a significant influence on the limit of what is considered "acceptable" rancidity. While food-grade oils have acceptable limits of rancidity not exceeding 2 meq/kg[10], GOED is currently upholding 5 meq/kg, making their standard more liberal. In a lot of studies, the mean of PV measurements (a measurement of rancidity) is exceeding the 2 meq/kg limit but stay within the GOED standard.

What Is Inside A Fish Oil Supplement?

Many fish oil supplements contain many more fatty acids than DHA and EPA. One study isolating fatty acids from the top 3 selling fish oil supplements found 30-plus different fatty acids, including 1/3 saturated fat. As expected, all three supplements had peroxides levels (rancidity values) higher than deemed acceptable[11]. In 2013, an investigation into fish oil in South Africa found that over 80% of the different brands had a higher quantity of peroxides than considered acceptable[12]. Before that, the same author concluded that the majority of the fish oil supplements contained conjugated diene (CD), as a marker of rancidity. The fish oils had more CD than vegetable oils that had been in open containers[13]. In 2015 in the United States, 117 fish oil supplements were measured, which showed that at least 50% of the supplements failed one of several tests[14]. The levels of these peroxides in human blood can predict disease and death in patients. The higher levels of peroxides, the worse the outcome of many pathologies[15], often independent of cholesterol levels[16].

Barry Halliwell, one of the most cited researchers in the world studying fish oil supplements, typically found amounts of 20-30% of lipid peroxides in fish oil supplements[17]. These lipid peroxides can be taken up just like non-oxidized fats and incorporated into the different lipoproteins[18]. These lipoproteins with oxidized fats can contribute to heart disease[19] and many other pathologies. The oxidation of fish oils into rancid and oxidative molecules is not something new or out of the norm: looking at cod liver oils (which have a high unsaturated fish oil content) in the 1930s in India, and it was found that 64% failed to meet requirements[20].

Who Is This Book For?

I write this book for people taking omega-3, thinking about taking omega-3, know someone who is taking omega-3, and anybody interested in an alternative health perspective. Until recently, only the positive sides of omega-3 have been popularized in the media. This book would like to make the case that a decrease in omega-6 would be healthier than an increase in omega-3. A deficiency in omega-3 that is sometimes observed could be an accumulation of omega-3 breakdown products, masking a deficiency, and potentially making conditions worse. When organisms age or are challenged by a stressor, their defensive mechanisms are decreased, and a significant decrease in DHA, EPA, and AA levels can be seen[21]. An increase in unsaturated breakdown products is found (malonaldehyde, dityrosine, neuroprostanes)[22].

What Are Omega-3 Fish Oils?

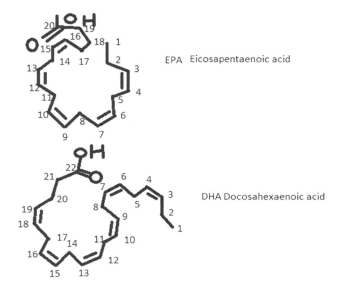

EPA Eicosapentaenoic acid

DHA Docosahexaenoic acid

Fats consist of carbon (numbered), hydrogen, and oxygen atoms. We can broadly divide fats into saturated and unsaturated. The saturated fats are linked by single bonds between the carbons (and are saturated with hydrogen). In contrast, unsaturated fats have one or more double bonds (2 linkages between the carbons, leaving less hydrogen attached to the carbon atom and considered unsaturated).

C-C-C-C-C-C-C-C-C-C-C-COOH =Saturated fat
C-C-C=C-C-C=C-C-C=C-C-C=C-C-C=C-C-C=C-C-C-COOH = Unsaturated fat

When the first double bond is 3 carbons from the methyl end, the fat is classified as an omega-3, while when the first omega is 6 carbons from the methyl end, we know it as an omega-6. There are several omega-3 fatty acids, and these can be classified by the number of double bonds and the total number of carbons.

C-C-C=C OMEGA-3
C-C-C-C-C-C=C OMEGA-6

Omega-3 and Omega-6 are deemed as essential, as the human body cannot make these fats endogenously (from within our own bodies). It is generally considered that in the Western diet, the consumption of omega-6 is too high. At the same time, the omega-3 intake is deemed insufficient. I would like to make the case that both omega-3 and omega-6 are potentially dangerous, and any increase in the consumption of these fats could have adverse consequences. When omega-6 is not excessive, "adequate" omega-3 fatty acids levels can be achieved with an average diet via the elongase and desaturase pathways[23].

Functions Of Omega-3

The primary fatty acids that are seen as fish oils are EPA and DHA. EPA is usually seen as healthy for joints and heart, while DHA is seen as necessary for eye and brain health. Omega-3 supplements typically consist of 18% EPA and 12% DHA. EPA is used up quicker than DHA, which has a longer-lasting function on average. From studying the literature, omega-3 seems to have a whole range of effects, which can be condensed into 3 main tasks.

1. Membrane, omega-3 can be incorporated into phospholipids and sphingolipids, which are part of the cell membrane. A phospholipid can consist of 2 fatty acids attached to a glycerol backbone, and the third position of the glycerol backbone is a phosphate with a head group. As with fish, the human membrane lipid consists mostly of the phosphatidylcholine form and is mainly in the SN-2 position (both omega-3 and

omega-6 compete for this position). The SN-1 position is usually saturated, while the phospholipid SN-3 position can be part of the membrane.

2. Energy Storage and Thermal Function, DHA, and EPA can be used for storage and insulation in fish. Still, the residues of fish oils in humans are thought to be less than the intake. However, rat studies show that fish oils are readily incorporated[24] within adipose tissue. It has been argued that EPA is readily mobilized from fat stores due to its double bonds near its ethyl ending. Omega-3 fats seem to be stored at a slow pace[25] and seem to favor the liver in phospholipids instead of adipose tissues[26]. The polyunsaturated are generally stored in the hips and buttocks and saturated fats in the abdominal area[27]. Fats can be used for energy production for the requirement of ATP. ATP is the way the cell gets energized. Studies show that EPA is being oxidized at a higher rate than DHA, which has a longer-lasting function.

3. Messaging Molecules, omega-3 can be part of an intercellular and extracellular messaging complex with a wide range of responses. We can convert the unsaturated fats into eicosanoids. These molecules have many functions in the body. The omega-3 and -6 have different messaging products and actions using the same enzymes. Omega-3 has a variety of responses with regards to enzyme activity within the cell and gene expression within the nucleus of the cell. EPA can be transformed into E resolvins, and DHA can be converted into D resolvins, marinsins, protectins, and neuroprotectins. These molecules can have useful actions, but unfortunately, these molecules are new, and all their potential effects have not been fully elucidated.

For example, resolvins D1 can increase nitric oxide and prostacyclin[28], and both molecules are known to have adverse effects.

Fish Oil Ingestion

Once fish oil is digested, the fats can be taken up in the gastrointestinal tract. In the tract, they are separated and transported into mixed micelles, then re-esterified in chylomicrons in which they are transported in the lymph system, before entering into the blood circulation. From the blood, the fish oils can be carried by albumin and can be released by lipases for tissue integration. Most of the fish oil is deposited in myocardial and retina, brain, and nervous tissue or used up for its different functions.

EPA Versus DHA

EPA can be converted into DHA but has its attributes. EPA has, in many ways, healthier functions than DHA. EPA has fewer double bonds than DHA, making EPA less fragile. Because of the similarity with the very inflammatory arachidonic acid (AA 20 carbon/omega-6), EPA can inhibit AA pathways that are known to be inflammatory. By competing for the same enzymes, EPA can inhibit the omega-6 pathways into eicosanoids. Because arachidonic acid is so prevalent in the Western diet and is beginning to be a "recognized" nutritional problem[29], stopping this fatty acid from becoming pro-inflammatory can be seen as healthy (additionally, aspirin works in the same way).

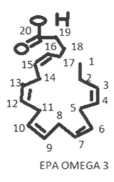
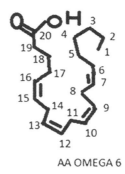

EPA OMEGA 3   AA OMEGA 6

Research And Commerce

The standards and parameters set on what is "good" and "healthy" food seem to be greatly influenced by political and economic criteria rather than scientific ones. Food nutrition research only really started in the mid-1930s, and guidelines were given along the lines of financial systems. Furthermore, most scientists at that time (and some still today) did not think of nutrition as a respectable science since nutrition and supplements were associated with 'snake-oil' salesmen. The onset of World War II brought tighter bonds between the existing food conglomerates, governments, and the different advisory committees that provided advice about the recommended intake of food and health[30].

"no tolerable upper intake level (UL) for EPA, DHA or DPA has been set by any authoritative body"[31]

Products, Nutrition. (2012). Scientific Opinion on the Tolerable Upper Intake Level of eicosapentaenoic acid (EPA), docosahexaenoic acid (DHA) and docosapentaenoic acid (DPA). EFSA Journal. 10. 10.2903/j. efsa. 2012. 2815.

This statement was made by the European Food Safety Authority (EFSA) in 2012. After reading the report, it becomes clear that the reason for this comment is due to the lack of information on the subject - not because the research showed its safety. This can also mean that fish oils are free to experiment with and are considered safe.

| Untapped Potential

Unsaturated fats, including DHA & EPA, have many effects on the body and are involved in many pathways and (de) activation of genes. This makes fish oils a promising agent for a scientist to make novel discoveries upon. In particular, fish oils, whose routes are still not fully elucidated, are a potential goldmine for getting one's name in the record books. Many of the leading science writers today writing about the benefits of omega-3 are in close contact with or have been paid by companies that have an interest in selling fish oil as part of their product. I am not suggesting a conspiracy, collusion, or even malicious intent. I am indicating that with an overemphasis of selected studies and a label of essentiality, fish oil has achieved an overall undeserved status as a miracle supplement. Fish oil studies are frequently financed by edible fat conglomerates or pharmaceutical companies[32][33], by scientists who are paid or employed by conglomerates and or pharmaceutical companies[34], or by governmental agencies that promote the use of fish oils. Conglomerates organize symposiums that are attended by international scientists and policymakers to enforce specific messages. These elected scientists, bureaucrats, and strategists work out a strategy to implement plans for "education" of scientists, hospitals, schools, and the community[35]. This top-down approach is potentially hazardous in science as it stifles independent thought and critique, as well as possibly having a definite financial motive. Some examples include:

- A 2003 study compared EPA and DHA (omega-3 fish oils) with ALA (omega-3 plant oil) and an omega-6 (plant oil) on atherosclerosis risk factors. One focus was the oxidation of LDL cholesterol, as oxidized LDL is a risk factor in heart disease. The results showed that increased oxidation of LDL was seen in the fish oil group, even though less fish oil was supplemented than the other oils in the other groups. The authors concluded that ALA and EPA/DHA have "different" effects instead of adverse impacts generated by fish oils[36].
- The pharmaceutical companies may support foundations that could finance research that puts omega-3 in a favorable light. Mead Johnson provides omega-3 fatty acids in infant formula. Mead Johnson supports the March of Dimes Foundation which, in turn, finances studies that may favor omega-3. A 2011 study concluded that supplementing DHA results in a decrease in colds, compared to a soy/corn oil placebo. Looking into the study, one finds that beyond decreased colds, the DHA group experienced a higher increase in rashes, longer duration of nasal congestion, and longer length of vomiting, which were not mentioned in the conclusion[37].
- No differences are found in depression treatment with DHA, EPA or placebo (soybean), but side-effects include 13,3% for EPA, 14,3% for DHA, but 0% in placebo for constipation and 1,7% EPA, 8,9% DHA and 0% for placebo for tremors. Even after one patient in the EPA group had to stop due to increased depression (the placebo group also had one person stop due to reactions to the placebo pill), it was concluded that EPA and DHA were well tolerated[38].
- In many studies, one can initially find that fish oils are well tolerated, only to see that if the placebo group (often with

other unsaturated oils) showed no differences. When fish oil showed adverse effects in 25% of test subjects and the placebo group has 23% with other fats, the study concludes that fish oils are well tolerated[39].

When the title states that the addition of saturated fatty acids to fish oil diet alters the inflammatory response in mice, one has to read the study to find out that saturated fatty acids decrease the inflammatory response from fish oil to stressors[40]. When olive oil outperforms fish oil and sunflower oil in tooth health, the title is stated as fish oil being equal to olive oil. When looking at the teeth and inspecting the bone loss figures, it was established that bone loss in the fish oil group was doubled compared to olive oil[41] (see picture below).

Bullon P, Battino M, Varela-Lopez A, Perez-Lopez P, Granados-Principal S, Ramirez-Tortosa MC, et al. (2013) Diets Based on Virgin Olive Oil or Fish Oil but Not on Sunflower Oil Prevent Age-Related Alveolar Bone Resorption by Mitochondrial-Related Mechanisms. PLoS ONE 8(9): e74234. https://doi.org/10.1371/journal.pone.0074234).

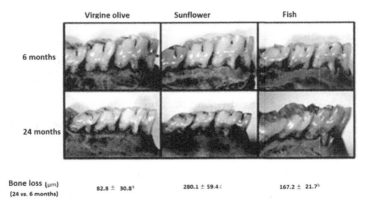

It is important to note that omega-3 can replace olive oil[424344] (and omega-6). This, by itself, is problematic as the ratio of monounsaturated to polyunsaturated fats (omega-6) is a significant indicator of LDL susceptibility (an indicator of heart disease). As the mono- to polyunsaturated ratio becomes lower, LDL particles become more susceptible to oxidation[45].

But I Thought That Omega-3 Were Healthy Oils?

Looking at the media, everybody knows that omega-3 fatty acids are healthy, almost everybody knows that saturated fats are bad. Many people know that people have a "deficiency" in omega-3. These claims are usually unopposed and exacerbated when yet another study has found that omega-3 has healthy properties/ effects. Although touted as miracle health supplements, Omega-3 supplementation has a lesser-known side to them. The speed with which fish oil could become rancid labeled them "perhaps" the most dangerous food in the world from a scientific perspective.

"From the angle of medical care and science, however, dead raw fish is perhaps the most dangerous kind of food that exist. The primary cause of death in fish is asphyxia and immediately after death the structure and composition of tissue changes"[46]

OBSERVATIONS ON THE BASIC NUTRITION, VITAMINS AND FOOD PREPARATIONS IN DOLPHINS. By C.F.G.W. van der Hurk, D.V.M., veterinary consultant to the Dolfinarium, Harderwijk, Bree 37, Rotterdam, Netherlands. Page 10 of the volume. Aquatic Mammals, Volume 1(2), 9-21. Permission from Aquatic Mammals Journal.

Omega-3 Supplement Sales And Requirements

Omega-3 fish oil sales increased to about 30 billion (USD)[47] in 2016 and ranked amongst the most popular supplements in the US[48][49].

Some scientists have wondered why fish oil supplementation has increased despite its ineffectiveness in research studies[50]. There have been over 23,000 research articles regarding fish oils and more than 2500 human trials. Recommended intake from the World Health Organization of omega-3 for the general population is about 1-2% of total caloric intake. The United States recognized up to 3 grams a day as safe in 1997. The National Institute of Health suggests an intake of above 1 gram per day; one serving of fatty fish is roughly within this range. This, by itself, can be problematic as studies with rats show that a 3% intake of fish oils have shown to cause lipid peroxidation (the breakdown of fats) in serum and tissues[51]. The average consumption of omega-3 from seafood is estimated at just above 160 mg/day (a slight increase from 1990)[52]. It is about the same for men and women. To illustrate that humans don't need more than the amount already consumed, one can look at the Maasai. The Maasai people living in Tanzania and Kenya live mostly on milk and plants. The EPA intake is estimated at 29 mg and DHA as low as 6 mg per day. Probably because their overall PUFA intake is low, their omega-3 blood levels are normal[53].

The precursor for fish oils is alpha-linolenic acid (ALA). ALA is found in vegetables and meat, and the average intake of ALA is thought to be 1.5 grams a day. This average 1.5 gram accounts for about 0.675% of energy intake (in a 2000 calorie diet) per day. Even without the fish intake, the ALA would be sufficient as studies with rats show that 0.5% of ALA energy intake sustained normal growth[54][55]. About 0.44% of it is seen as a minimal requirement for patient care[56]. An increase in ALA does not consistently increase DHA. When 1.2 grams per day was given to volunteers, after 12 weeks, DHA content in the erythrocyte membrane was the same as when subjects were given 3.6 grams of ALA per day[57].

Fish Oil Is Processed Food

"Although the refining process has been studied for several years, many of the investigations are still directed towards oils of vegetable origin, which involves the evaluation of several stages and new techniques that have not yet been reported for fish oil"[58]

Bonilla-Méndez, J. R., & Hoyos-Concha, J. L. (2018). Methods of extraction, refining and concentration of fish oil as a source of omega-3 fatty acids. Permission from Ciencia y TecnologíaAgropecuaria, 19 (3), 645-668. https://doi.org/10.21930/rcta.vol19_num2_art:684

Fish oil is manufactured on a grand scale, and the manufacturing is a lengthy process. Although there are different ways to "make" fish oil, the procedure usually consists of the following aspects[59][60][61][62].

10 Steps For Making Fish Oil

1. **Settling/Degumming** (making the oil stand, this can include heating the oil and adding acids to separate the oil from the water. This phase also includes squeezing the fats out of the protein)
2. **Deacidification** (adding alkali to de-acidify, possibly leading to resin)
3. **Bleaching** (The oil get heated to 80 degree Celsius while bleaching clay is added to remove pigments and soaps)
4. **Deodorisation** (free fatty acids, ketones and aldehydes are removed by several mechanisms)
5. **Storage and Anti-oxidants**
6. **Refining of Oil**
7. **Deacidification and trans-esterification** (separating the fats into fatty acids, usually under high temperatures of above 80 degree Celsius)
8. **Molecular Distillation** (a technique that purifies and concentrates the fatty acids, the temperature can go up to 150 degree Celsius)
9. **Deodorisation** (fatty acids are combined with bleaching clay and/or activated carbon to remove impurities. The temperature can go up to 85 degree Celsius)
10. **Antioxidants**

Newer techniques include ultrasounds-assisted (UAE) and supercritical fluid extraction (SFE). These techniques allow for lower temperatures.

From ALA To DHA

Humans can convert the different omega-3 fatty acids into other omega-3 fatty acids via elongase enzymes that add carbons and desaturase enzymes that attach double bonds to the fatty acid. The omega-3 and -6 use the same proteins/enzymes and compete.

18:3 Alpha-Linolenic Acid
Delta-6-Desaturase
18:4 Octadecatetraenoic Acid
Elongase
20:4 Eicosatetraenoic Acid
Delta-5-Desaturase
20:5 Eicosapentaenoic Acid (EPA)
F3 Isoprostanes, Resolvins, Hydroxyl Fatty Acids, Leukotrienes, Prostanoids
Elongase
22:5 Docosapentaenoic : Hydroxy Fatty Acids
Elongase
24:5 Tetracosapentaneoic Acid
Delta-4-Desaturase
24:6 Tetracosahexaeoic Acid
Beta-Oxidation
Docosahexaenoic Acid (DHA) F4 Isoprostanes, Resolvins, Protectins, Maresins, Fatty Acids
*There are minor pathways in which DHA can be reconstituted into EPA

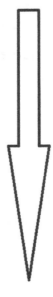

Making Fats Shorter Or Larger

The different Fats

Enzymes that make fats more unsaturated

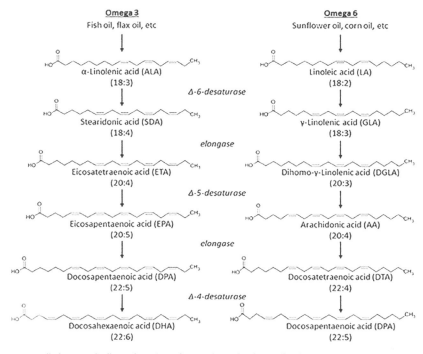

From: Elinder F and Liin SI (2017) Actions and Mechanisms of Polyunsaturated Fatty Acids on Voltage-Gated Ion Channels. Front. Physiol. 8:43. doi: 10.3389/fphys.2017.00043

What Are Fish Oils In This Book?

Within this book, EPA and DHA are the two fatty acids that are used to classify fish oil. Fish contains many fats, but have an increased amount of EPA and DHA compared to other animals. Fish oils are usually stored in a glycerol formation. The glycerol bond has, depending on the function, 2 or 3 fatty acids attached to the glycerol. These 2 or 3 fatty acids can be saturated, unsaturated, or a combination of the two.

GLYCEROL

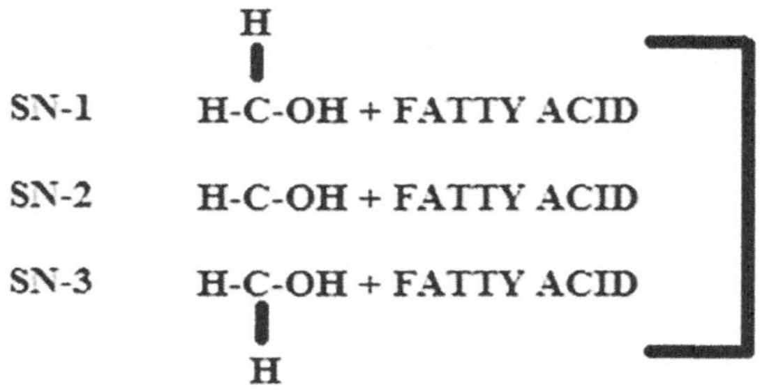

$$\begin{array}{ll}
 & H \\
 & | \\
\text{SN-1} & H\text{-}C\text{-}OH + FATTY\ ACID \\
 & \\
\text{SN-2} & H\text{-}C\text{-}OH + FATTY\ ACID \\
 & \\
\text{SN-3} & H\text{-}C\text{-}OH + FATTY\ ACID \\
 & | \\
 & H
\end{array}$$

stereospecific numbering (sn)

The unsaturated fat is usually in the SN-2 position, probably for protective reasons, as if fish oil is attached to either SN-1 or SN-3, it becomes more prone to be oxidized[63]. When a fatty acid gets released from the glycerol bond, it becomes a free fatty acid. Free fatty acids are usually increased in stressful conditions.

TAG Or EE

Per year, the global production of fish oil is about 1,000,000 tonnes. They use most of this for nutrition. Fish oil in fish is usually found in the form of triacylglycerols (TAG). It contains little or no ethyl esters (EE), while ethyl esters and TAG are sold in supplements. Ethyl esters are fragile and easy to oxidize, while TAG is more stable and could be seen as safer. Because fish oils in their natural state are high in saturated fats (30%), triacylglycerols are esterified into free fatty acids. The unsaturated fats (DHA & EPA) are isolated, and because of the high cost of re-esterified (back into the more stable

TAG), usually, ethyl esters are sold as fish oils. These EE is more vulnerable than TAG, and therefore potentially more harmful. The fish oils that are sold on the market usually do not state whether the oils are in TAG or EE form[64].

Problems With Fish Oils Research

Fish oil is still in the beginning stage of research compared to omega-6. Sometimes the controls are being fed omega-6[656667], which has many ill effects on the body. The total quantities of omega-3 consumed compared to omega-6, and saturated fats are very low, making its impacts on the body challenging to measure. EPA and DHA seem to be too fragile to be fully metabolized[68], and it has been shown that many of the unsaturated fats do not reach the lymphatic system, and its toxicity occurs in the intestines[69]. Some studies with fish oils that have unfavorable results are not published. When, for example, feeding livestock fishmeal's findings are not useful for increasing growth and or offspring, the researchers can decide not to publish (mentioned in[70]). When fish oils are presented to animals for scientific research, it often results in reduced intake or rejection of fish oils[7172].

"The feeding of fish oil, however, frequently led to reduced food acceptance or rejection, and to histopathological changes in the liver"[73]

Verschuren PM, Houtsmuller UM, Zevenbergen JL. Evaluation of vitamin E requirement and food palatability in rabbits fed a purified diet with a high fish oil content. Lab Anim. 1990;24(2):164–171. Permission from SAGE Journals doi:10.1258/002367790780890167

The odor and taste could be responsible for this reduced intake. Reduced food consumption can have profound health-promoting effects, as seen in chronically restricted diets[74]. From a historical perspective, fish oil intake was so small compared to omega-6 that it was not a priority to investigate[75]. The fish oils used in medical experiments are kept under medical conditions. These conditions are not your typical fridge conditions but are held under N-2 at -20 degrees[76]. Because fish oil oxidizes so quickly, it is difficult to measure the right quantities of omega-3 that are fully assimilated[777879].

Short-term Solution

Short-term fish oil supplementation can be helpful as it can suppress the production of antibodies and other immune cells. It can upregulate defensive molecules like glutathione by lipid peroxidation. Many studies only show these short-term positive actions, leaving out its possible long-term disadvantages. When rats are fed fish, sunflower, or olive oil for a long duration (24 months), olive oil outperforms both fish and sunflower oils concerning liver health. While sunflower showed fibrosis, increased breakdown of fats, and fewer mitochondria, fish oil also showed more breakdown of fats and fewer mitochondria and less energy production by interfering with the electron transport chain[80].

Vitamin E And Fish Oil

"Furthermore, rats co-supplemented with fish oil and vitamin E exhibited significant decreases in both lipid peroxidation and protein oxidation levels in both liver and muscle"[81]

Patel BP, Safdar A, Raha S, Tarnopolsky MA, Hamadeh MJ (2010) Caloric Restriction Shortens Lifespan through an Increase in Lipid Peroxidation,

Inflammation and Apoptosis in the G93A Mouse, an Animal Model of ALS. PLoS ONE 5 (2): e9386. https://doi.org/10.1371/journal.pone.0009386

It is rare to find fish oils that do not have vitamin E added to them. Many studies have found that vitamin E added to fish oils could be more helpful than the fish oils themselves[82]. Vitamin E is used to keep the oxidation of fish oils in check and is known as a chain breaker. Eventually, fish oil oxidation can overwhelm the antioxidant system, resulting in unchecked inflammatory processes. Fish oil is so fragile that it can break down into smaller molecules that can be very harmful. One of the most frequent methods used to measure these smaller molecules is called TBARS (ThioBarbituric Acid Reactive Substances), which looks for dangerous particles. The way vitamin E interacts with fish oils can lead to a decrease in vitamin E levels. A reduction of vitamin E can have serious health consequences. One study found that after following 102 healthy persons older than 80 years for almost four years, 32 cardiovascular events were noted. Vitamin E was found to be critical as the elderly with the highest vitamin E had a 1/6 chance of cardiovascular events compared to those persons with the lowest amount of vitamin E. Lipid peroxidation was inversely associated with vitamin E. The group with the highest peroxidation levels had a 7-fold chance of heart disease compared with the lowest lipid peroxidation. Cholesterol had no significant association[83].

"Additionally, the n-3 fatty acids in fish oil are highly polyunsaturated and are therefore more readily oxidized, leading to higher lipid peroxidation"[84]

Patel BP, Safdar A, Raha S, Tarnopolsky MA, Hamadeh MJ (2010) Caloric Restriction Shortens Lifespan through an Increase in Lipid Peroxidation, Inflammation and Apoptosis in the G93A Mouse, an Animal Model of ALS. PLoS ONE 5 (2): e9386. https://doi. org/10.1371/journal.pone.0009386

PUFA And Vitamin E

As the amount of PUFA intake has been increasing over the last century (277%), the increase in vitamin E intake has lagged (249%). This lagging of vitamin E becomes more critical as one understands that as PUFA increases, the need for vitamin E goes up with each double bond instead of standardizing for grams per fat. Fish oils, which have 5 and 6 double bonds with EPA and DHA, will increase the need for vitamin E even if the total intake of fat stays the same (substituted for other fats). The vitamin E recommendations that are mostly in use today originate from the 1960s and do not account for a per double bond basis. This requirement is based on the 1960 typical diet and consists of 0.6 milligrams (mg) of vitamin E to every gram of unsaturated fat. In fact, in the 1960s, it was already established that this recommendation is not far from one obtaining vitamin E deficiency symptoms[85]. The 0.6 mg of vitamin E was found to be a minimal intake, not as an absolute requirement. It was suggested that if the total PUFA was low, vitamin E could also be lower than 0.6 mg. This 0.6 mg of vitamin E per 1 gram polyunsaturated is still in use today as a general rule. This does not take into account that more double bonds require more vitamin E. In farming and animal feeding, the vitamin E requirements were more specific, considering the double bonds per fatty acid. This requirement is entirely different, in which 1 gram of oleic acid requires 0.13 IU/G 1 double bonds vs. DHA is 2.70 IU/G 6 double bonds[86]. Beyond the limited intake of vitamin E, the PUFA itself impairs the absorption of vitamin E from the intestine (probably by the destruction of tocopherol by lipid peroxidation[87][88]). This is problematic because people consume most tocopherol together with the ingestion of PUFA (as with fish oil), which is already limited[89]. Most studies use the plasma test, which is cheap but may not be very useful. The ratio of lipid-adjusted plasma a-tocopherol could be more helpful. Where only 1-2% of an elderly population was vitamin E deficient according to plasma test, which tests the ratio of plasma tocopherol to lipids, 12% of the same communities had low tocopherol levels according to lipid-adjusted tocopherol to plasma lipids[90].

The Holy Omega-3 / Omega-6 Ratio

Omega-3, together with the omega-6, are seen as the essential fatty acids (EFA). The principal reason fish oils could be supplemented was to combat the enormous quantity of unsaturated vegetable oils (omega-6) that flooded the market after World War II. The increase in vegetable oil came about after the association was made between saturated fat and the increases in cholesterol. Vegetable oil is loaded with omega-6 and resulted in a significant discrepancy between the intake of omega-3 and omega-6. Instead of correcting the initial problem of limiting unsaturated fats by restricting omega-6, increasing omega-3 can likely increase many of the existing problems. The importance of the ratio of omega-3 to omega-6 is often suggested and has become a credo. This observation can often be seen in a different light. When looking at total PUFA quantities, a similar view can be observed. When people with venous thromboembolism are compared with a control group, a higher ratio of omega-6 to omega-3 is seen, but also a lower total PUFA content (controls have more elevated cholesterol)[91].

The same is observed for glaucoma, where fish oil is associated with a lower risk of glaucoma; the same association, however, can be made for lower PUFA intake (again, cholesterol is slightly higher in the control group)[92]. The graph below shows the number of double bonds per age group. When fatty acid content of blood cell membranes of older people is compared for fatty acids with younger age groups, omega-3 is higher in the oldest group (100 years +), but overall PUFA is amongst the lowest. Overall, the oldest age group resembles the youngest age group.

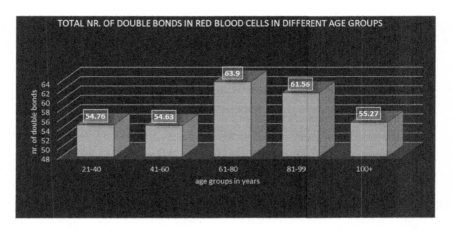

Data taken from [93] Rabini RA, Moretti, N, Staffolani R, et al. Reduced susceptibility to peroxidation of erythrocyte plasma membranes from centenarians. Exp Gerontol. 2002;37(5):657-663. doi:10.1016/s0531-5565(02)00006-2

Examples Of Why The Omega-3/Omega-6 Ratios May Not Be Useful

- When the fish oils are supplemented in different ratios to lower the ratio of omega-6 to omega-3, the results surprised the scientists. Three groups fed the ratio's omega-6 to omega-3 were, in group 1 (31:1), group 2, (5.4:1), and group 3 (1.4:1) in old dogs. The results showed that the dogs displayed a reduced cell-mediated immune response, showed increase breakdown products of fats, and a lowered vitamin E quantity in the lowered omega-6 to omega-3 ratio[94].

- They can insert a gene into mice to change omega-6 into omega-3 to increase the ratio between omega-3 and omega-6. These mice can be compared to a control group and other groups that lack this gene. Results show that when tested on non-alcohol fatty liver disease, the omega-3 increased group had the greatest liver damage and the most significant increase in fat accumulation of all groups. These gene-inserted mice had omega-3 to omega-6 ratio of about 1 to 1[95]. The results made the scientists suggest to caution fish oil use for NASH patients (non-alcoholic steatohepatitis).
- When young chickens are separated into six groups, each on different diets that affect the ratio between omega-3 and omega-6, it was shown that higher omega-3 (while leaving total PUFA the same) resulted in increased DNA damage and overall increased lipid peroxidation[96].
- When overall PUFA levels are higher but have a lower ratio of omega-3 to omega-6, it does not translate into better health. Children with recently diagnosed diabetes and established diabetes have higher omega-3 quantities and a lower omega-3 to omega-6 ratio than healthy controls[97].
- In one group, slightly more omega-3 (EPA) are given than omega-6 at a ratio of 1.24 to 1.0 (omega-3 to omega-6) and compared to diets comprising of omega-6 to omega-3, 9 to 1.0 and 7.6 to 1.0 in mice to assess liver injury in paracetamol feeding. After examining the livers of the three groups, it was found that the EPA group had the highest amount of liver injury and inflammatory gene responses[98].
- When pregnant rats are fed an increased amount of omega-3, resulting in a ratio of omega-3 to omega-6 from

4.8 compared to 8.4 in the control group, the offspring shows increased total fat deposits and subcutaneous fat mass. In contrast, the control had normal fat levels[99].

One team of researchers noted the mutagenicity (cancer-causing ability) of fish oil in combination with omega-6. They wrote;

"A recent trend of balancing high ω-6 intake in modern diet with increased ω-3 consumption can prove futile if one considers the ω-3 PUFAs as initiators and ω-6 PUFAs as promoters of cancer"[100]

Grúz, Petr & Shimizu, Masatomi & Sugiyama, Kei-Ichi & Honma, Masamitsu. (2017). Mutagenicity of ω-3 fatty acid peroxidation products in the Ames test. Mutation Research/Genetic Toxicology and Environmental Mutagenesis. 819. 10.1016/j. mrgentox. 2017. 05. 004

There are many ways in which fish oil can be involved in the initiation and progression of cancer. One way is its immunosuppression quality, as immunosuppressive conditions can lead to an increase and initiator of cancer[101][102]. Another way in which fish oil can be involved in cancer is through its breakdown products. Fish oils can break down into the α (alpha) - and β (beta) -unsaturated aldehydes. These α and β-unsaturated aldehydes can link with the bases of DNA and form adducts with DNA, possibly leading to cancer and potentially many other pathologies. As one study observed:

"Particularly damaging, ROS can initiate a free radical chain-reaction in unsaturated fatty acids, thereby generating toxic electrophilic α/β unsaturated aldehydes, a process called lipid peroxidation. The best characterized of these carbonyl-derivatives are 4-hydroxy-2-nonenal (4-HNE), malondialdehyde (MDA) and acrolein"[103]

Petersen DR, Saba LM, Sayin VI, Papagiannakopoulos T, Schmidt EE, Merrill GF, et al. (2018) Elevated Nrf-2 responses are insufficient to mitigate protein carbonylation in hepatospecific PTEN deletion mice. PLoS ONE 13 (5): e0198139. https://doi.org/10.1371/journal.pone.0198139

I think overall these symptoms - decreased immune response, dangerous messaging molecules, and total increased breakdown products - are the major worries when speaking of adverse fish oil effects. Despite many articles showing otherwise, there seems to be a decrease in the ratio of omega-6 and omega-3 in the last 40 years (USA data[104]). As two scientists argued back in 2011, the low status of omega-3 is not because of low omega-3 intake, and it is likely because of the enormous increase in omega-6[105].

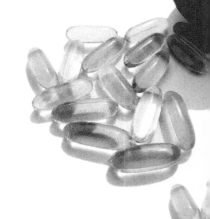

CHAPTER 2

Fish Oil Versus Fish

"One limitation of some of these studies has been the lack of distinction between fatty and lean fish"[106]

Rylander C, Sandanger TM, Engeset D, Lund E (2014) Consumption of Lean Fish Reduces the Risk of Type 2 Diabetes Mellitus: A Prospective Population Based Cohort Study of Norwegian Women. PLoS ONE 9 (2): e89845. https://doi.org/10.1371/journal.pone.0089845

To focus on fish oil, one has to exclude all other nutrients present in fish. Fish contains many nutrients in significant quantities and can be a part of a healthy diet by itself. Many of the studies that put fish oil in a favorable light were conducted with fish-eating populations. These studies were associated with fish oil but could have readily been associated with the other nutrients in fish or the substitution of other foods that were excluded while eating fish. While consuming fish is associated with later onset of brain impairments, fish oils are not[107]. The intake of non-fried fish is related to a decrease in mortality. At the same time, high omega-3 consumption is associated with an increase in mortality, compared to lower omega-3 consumption[108]. Alpha-synuclein is seen as one of the prime contributors to Parkinson's disease and can be increased by fish oil. Beta-parvalbumin is a protein that is readily available in fish and can inhibit alpha-synuclein, making this fish protein protective against fish oil peroxidation[109].

The complete package of fish is likely very anti-inflammatory. The nutritional content of fish keeps the potentially dangerous fats in fish in check. This lack of proteins, minerals, and vitamins is probably the reason that the omega-3 is incorporated into the human body at a 2- to 9-fold lower rate via supplements than through fish intake[110]. I would like to examine some molecules present in fish and are potentially being confused with fish oils.

Cod Liver Oil

One problem with researching omega-3 is that cod liver oil is often supplemented as omega-3[111][112]. Cod liver oil has a lengthy history of treating different kinds of illnesses. Fish liver oil and livers from mammals have been used before the time of the Vikings (they used to mix milk with cod liver oil)[113]. From the writings of Hippocrates and Pliny, we know that the oils of dolphins were used for skin conditions. In 1789, the English doctor Darbey mentioned cod liver oil as having a curative effect on rheumatics. A century later, Dutch fishermen found that cod liver oils would cure rickets in some conditions[114]. From the 1880s until the 1940s, cod liver oil became a popular vitamin supplement. Of all fish liver oils, the cod liver was thought to have the highest amount of vitamin A and became popular (Many other fish livers have since been found to have higher amounts of vitamin A, notably whale, shark, herring, and swordfish liver[115][116]). This occurred until studies in the 1920s started showed the toxic effects of cod liver oil on different animals[117][118]. These included loss of vitamin E, heart lesions, muscular dystrophy, and eventual death[119]. The toxic effects were found not to be caused by the overload of vitamins A and D. They were found to be counteracted by vitamin B (brewer's yeast)[120] . The hydrogenation of the fats (making them less unsaturated) made them safer.

The research continued into the 1940s when researchers found that the unsaturated fats in fish liver oil were prone to oxidize and increase lipid peroxidation. The unsaturated fish liver oils contained less vitamin A[121] after peroxidation. The significance of rancid fats became substantial as the research developed. In the 1940s, it was known that unsaturated fats could inactivate vitamin D, vitamin E, and biotin (vitamin E protected biotin to some extent[122]). They also found the unsaturated fats in cod liver oil were also found to stain teeth[123]. When omega-3 is concentrated from cod liver oil, the harmful lipid oxidizing substances are numerous[124].

Taurine

Taurine is an amino acid (part of a protein) that has many effects in the body that omega-3 is thought to cause.

Taurine	Attributed to fish oils
Heart protective[125]	Heart protective
Abundant in the developing brain[126]	Abundant in the developing brain
Anti-inflammatory[127]	Anti-inflammatory
Increase HDL[128]	Increase HDL
Regulates blood pressure[129]	Regulates blood pressure
Normalize hypercholesteremia by increased cholesterol degradation, decrease LDL[130][131]	Lowers cholesterol levels, decrease LDL
Is mostly found in seafood, not a lot in land animal[132]	Is mostly found in seafood, not a lot in land animal
Increase cell membrane fluidity[133]	Increase cell membrane fluidity

Neuroprotective[134]	Neuroprotective

Selenium

Selenium is another mineral present at high levels in fish. Selenium is an essential mineral. Apart from its need to make amino acids, selenium can prevent lipid peroxidation[135]. Selenium is part of the detoxifying system glutathione peroxidase and, in parts, regulates its activity[136]. The decrease of glutathione can upregulate lipid peroxidation[137] and can result in a loss of selenium. Selenium can be released from the glutathione peroxidation molecule by loss of integrity caused by fish oil supplementation. It has been suggested to check for selenium deficiency when fish oils are supplemented[138]. As expected, a decline or decrease in cognitive functions is seen in the elderly with selenium deficiency[139].

Furan Fatty Acids

Furan fatty acids are fatty acids present in fish that have anti-inflammatory properties. These anti-inflammatory properties of furan acids seem to be more significant than those of EPA and inhibit lipid peroxidation[140]. These fatty acids are present in fish oils and could be responsible for possible positive outcomes[141]. Furan fatty acids are difficult to identify and isolate from fish oil supplements, making it challenging to study fish oil in isolation.

Fatty Fish Versus Lean Fish

Some advantages of fish, apart from the oil, can be seen when we compare fatty fish to lean fish. The leaner fish are often found in the more tropical seas, compared to the colder seas that harbor the oily fish. They found it that lean fish can lower blood pressure, while oily fish did not[142]. In adjusted models, lean fish consumption and not fatty fish consumption was associated with a decreased risk of having metabolic syndrome[143]. Although omega-3 is associated with fewer preterm pregnancies, the association with fewer preterm pregnancies is higher with lean fish than with the fatty fish[144]. Furthermore, lean fish was associated with a decrease in waist circumference. In contrast, oily fish was associated with an increase in waist circumference[145]. Lean fish have fewer vitamins than salmon. For example, oily fish is usually superior in vitamins B12, niacin, vitamin E, vitamin A, vitamin D, and vitamin B6[146]. The positive effects on plasma triacylglycerol (TAG) of lean fish (cod) are the same as when compared to fatty fish (salmon)[147].

	TOTAL FISH FAT	Percentages of fish oils (DHA, EPA)	Total fish oils (DHA, EPA) Gram
LEAN FISH			
COD	0.6	38.3	0.23
HADDOCK	1.0	34	0.34
FATTY FISH			
SALMON	10.0	24.5	2.45
MACKEREL	24.4	18.2	4.44
HERRING SUMMER	14.5	12.6	1.82
HERRING WINTER	19.0	24.8	4.72

148

As seen in the table, although the percentages of the lean fish can be higher (some lean fish like tusk and coalfish contain no omega-3), the total amount in grams is about tenfold the amount of omega-3 in favor of fatty fish. It is interesting to note that oily fish high in EPA and DHA naturally also contain the saturated fats myristic and palmitic acid, possibly as protective agents. Furthermore, in the winter and cold temperatures DHA and EPA can be stored in fatty acids, while in summer and warmer temperatures, these fatty acids are usually membrane-bound. The places where fish hold oxygen (in the swim bladder) does not contain any mitochondria, which are very susceptible to oxygen attack[149]. Both fatty and lean fish are associated with better cognitive performances[150], making the omega-3 cognitive increasing abilities less probable.

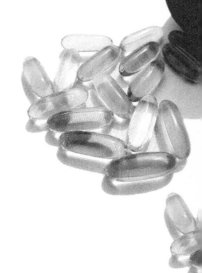

CHAPTER 3

The Nature Of Omega-3

Unsaturated Versus Saturated

"Animals fed diets containing relatively more polyunsaturated fatty acids 1) are more likely to hibernate, 2) hibernate earlier in the season, 3) have lower body temperatures / metabolic rates during torpor, and 4) have longer bouts of torpor than those given diets with lower levels of polyunsaturated fatty acids."[151]

Reproduced from 49 words. Craig L. Frank et al. The relationship between lipid peroxidation, hibernation, and food selection in mammals. Integrative & Comparative Biology (1998) 38 (2): 341-349. By permission of Oxford University Press on behalf of Society for Integrative and Comparative Biology. Available at: https://academic.oup.com/icb/article/38/2/341/213970?searchresult=1.

To better understand fish oils and unsaturated fats, it could be essential to look at temperature and hibernation. The unsaturation of fatty acids can be increased or decreased under certain conditions (more double bonds). The polyunsaturated fatty acids (PUFA) are predominately found in cold climates and seem to be a requirement for hibernation and/or for cold-blooded animals to survive. When you keep butter or coconut oil in your fridge, it stays solid, but fish oil will always remain liquid until well below freezing, making it essential for organisms with low body temperatures. The bends that the unsaturated fats have, make it difficult to pack tight and stay more fluid even in freezing temperatures. Fish containing omega-3 are mostly cold-blooded and reside in cold or arctic waters, whereas fish in tropical temperatures have less omega-3[152]. Unsaturated fats versus saturated show that unsaturated fats prolong hibernation. In contrast, saturated fats increase activity temperature and reduced fat stores[153].

Mitochondria

Mitochondria are seen as the batteries of the cell and provide energy and heat for the cell to thrive and maintain functions. When these mitochondria contain an excess of unsaturated fats, energy and heat are decreased. When comparing the tropical fats (saturated) with fish oils (unsaturated), it was found that fish oils showed reduced mitochondria function[154]. Even fish fed omega-3 revealed reduced activity of cytochrome c[155] (which is critical for proper respiration at the mitochondria).

The prominent researcher Lehninger, in the 1950s and 1960s, found that the longer unsaturated fatty acids caused swelling of the mitochondria, which could be restored by adding ATP. Lehninger suggested that unsaturated fats result in peroxidation and reduced glutathione levels, leading to swelling. He also found that aging mitochondria were less prone to respond to swelling and thus became desensitized. Recent studies show that the loss of the mitochondria membrane potential causes swelling of mitochondria, as well as impaired ATP production[156].

Although omega-3 intakes are limited compared to the omega-6, for hibernation in animals to occur, unsaturated fatty acids (n-3 & n-6) increase in the mitochondria and the adipose tissue[157]. Both moderate to high levels of DHA and EPA are shown to inhibit Na, K-ATPase activity, which is necessary to maintain proper mineral balance[158][159]. At the same time, vitamin E can prevent the loss of this function[160]. There have been many studies showing that fish oil decreases mitochondrial function and, additionally, a decrease in metabolic rate[161].

Some examples include

- When DHA is incorporated into the mitochondria, it decreases enzymatic activities compared to 18:2, omega-6[162]. This feature of reduced function of mitochondria is often observed when there is an accumulation of unsaturated fats in the mitochondria[163].
- Compared to olive oil (monounsaturated), fish oils will reduce Co2 production and thermogenesis[164][165]. Mitochondria enzymes are reduced with fish oil compared to safflower[166]. Compared to soy oil, fish oil decreases metabolic heat in organisms[167].
- Compared to the omega-6 rich corn oil, fish oil oxygen consumption is reduced via reduced cytochrome C[168]. Compared to coconut oil, the TTC mitochondrial tricarboxylate carrier is reduced on fish oils[169], as is seen in hypothyroidism[170] and starvation[171].
- Fish oil is known to reduce heart rate[172][173] and is associated with lower body temperature[174].

Cardiolipin

One of the unique and essential parts of the mitochondria is cardiolipin. Cardiolipin differs from other phospholipids and has several unique features. Cardiolipin is attached to many of the complexes (complex I, III, IV, V, and cytochrome C) that generate ATP, produce CO_2, and keep the cell energized. When DHA gets incorporated into cardiolipin, the binding of complexes within the mitochondria becomes disrupted and results in reduced mitochondria function even when compared to linoleic acid. After reintroducing linoleic acid, the mitochondria function is restored[175]. High fish intake can cause lower cardiolipin content[176]. In normal conditions, cardiolipin does not contain long unsaturated fatty acids like AA & DHA. These changes seem to occur in aging populations and pathologies[177][178]. DHA remodeling was recently observed when comparing healthy cardiac tissue with diabetes tissue, in which DHA levels among the diabetes patients were significantly higher[179]. *Furthermore, DHA can increase lipid peroxidation, which can lead to loss of cytochrome C leading to mitochondria dysfunction[180][181].*

Thyroid, Cardiolipin, And Fish Oil

Cardiolipin synthesis seems to be mainly regulated by thyroid hormone(s). When thyroid function is high, cardiolipin synthesis is increased, and when thyroid function is decreased, cardiolipin synthesis decreases[182][183]. The thyroid works, in many ways, in the opposite direction to the unsaturated fatty acids. As thyroid increases heat, PUFA tends to reduce it. In hypothyroid conditions, unsaturated fats tend to be made, while a high thyroid function favors the creation of saturated fats or the omega-9 fatty acids. Both saturated fats and omega-9 fatty acids are more resistant to heat and light. Fish oil has a limited role concerning thyroid health as it protects against the anti-thyroid actions of omega-6, but seem to have many anti-thyroid effects by itself. From studies with rats, we can see that fish oils can decrease both T4 (thyroxine) and the active T3 hormone (triiodothyronine)[184]. Fish oil in the bloodstream as non-esterified unsaturated fatty acids inhibit the binding of T4 to thyroxine-binding globulin. At the same time, saturated fats were found to be inactive[185][186]. After the thyroid is removed, the shorter fatty acid makes place for the longer fatty acids[187].

Many studies found that the unsaturated fatty acid inhibits the binding of thyroid hormone; these unsaturated increase their thyroid-inhibiting abilities as the fats have more double bonds[188]. Studies have found that unsaturated fats are uniquely suppressive of thyroid function through inhibiting the actions of the active thyroid hormone[189]. Polyunsaturated fats (mostly omega-6) have been used by the Agrarian Industry since the 1950s to fatten the animals by lowering their thyroid function - one researcher noted to improve stock conditions by:

"feeding them anti-thyroid drugs such as high levels of polyunsaturated fatty acids in diets."[190]

Scheele, Cor W. Ascites in chickens : oxygen consumption and requirement related to its occurrence / Cor W. Scheele - [S.l.: s.n.] Thesis Landbouwuniversiteit Wageningen. - With réf. - With summary in Dutch. ISBN 90-5485-499-5

Fish oil can increase T4, while leaving T3 the same, possibly increasing the RT3 (anti-thyroid hormone)[191]. The ease with which the unsaturated fats break down and increase reactive oxygen species can quickly decrease thyroid function. For example, increased lipid peroxidation and lowering of T3 are associated with spontaneous abortions[192].

Factors That Increase Unsaturation

An increase of darkness, estrogen, and coldness are three factors that increase during the start of hibernation. Thyroid hormone is, logically, reduced during hibernation, and mammals appear to become hypothyroid and change from glucose to fatty acid oxidation[193]. Overall, there is a decrease in energy by lowering the mitochondria function.

Certain factors increase unsaturated fats. These factors applied to the human body typically increase lipid peroxidation (non-enzymatic breakdown). Of all factors, coldness, darkness, and estrogen seem to have a significant influence. *Alternatively, heat, light, and androgens are associated with the formation of more saturated fats and a high metabolic rate.*

Coldness

Coldness can increase hypothyroidism[194] with lower thyroid hormones and function in the winter and higher values in the summer[195]. It has been shown that a cold climate increases the trend of making fats more unsaturated (ALA-EPA-DHA)[196]. Coldness increases the activity of the enzymes that add a bond to the unsaturation (delta- 6 – desaturase) growing from ALA (18:3n-3 to 18:4n-3) to ultimately DHA by the enzyme delta- 4-desaturase. Cells are thought to function optimally when they are within a specific range of membrane fluidity. During a decrease in temperature, genes for desaturase can be activated to accommodate[197].

Darkness

Light seems to inhibit the desaturase enzymes[198], and low light stimulates the conversion to increase unsaturation[199]. The thyroid hormone is down-regulated during long nights and winter. Conversely, lipid peroxidation is highest during the night (darkness)[200201202] and winter[203].

Most deaths occur in the early morning when estrogen and cortisol are high[204]. When rats are followed during the day and night cycles, lipid peroxidation is the highest between 20:00 and 04:00 hours. It was also observed that at this time, the PUFA content is the highest in parts of the brain[205206].

Estrogen

In bears, during hibernation, the ratio of estrogen to testosterone is 26 pg/ml to 1 ng/ml to about 2 pg/ml to 1 ng/ml in the summer. This same shift, although not this pronounced, is observed in humans when in the summer, estrogen is lower, and androgens are the same or higher. In winter, estrogen goes up and androgen decreases[207208]. Besides some nutritional deficiencies, darkness, and coldness, estrogen also speeds up the conversion of ALA to EPA and DHA (estrogen seems to favor omega-3 versus omega-6). Estrogen increases the activity of delta-5 and delta-6 desaturase enzymes[209210]. At the same time, progesterone does not affect the rate and testosterone decreased the conversion rate[211]. When testosterone decreases, lipofuscin (age spots), seems to increase[212]; fish oil is associated with lower testosterone levels[213].

The depressing action of testosterone on delta-5 and delta-6 desaturase was accompanied by an increase in delta-9-desaturase[214] (as is seen with the active thyroid hormone[215]). Although estrogen blood levels are sometimes associated with negative and sometimes positive outcomes, when the estrogen concentration is high in tissue, the results seem to be always negative[216][217][218][219]. The quantity of estrogen in postmenopausal women's tissues can be 50 times higher than blood serum levels and having little relation with each other, making blood tests not very useful[220]. *The unsaturated fats that the body makes itself have fewer double bonds and are more resistant to stress and the temperature of the human body.*

Estrogen increases the unsaturation of fatty acids, and unsaturated fats increase the release of estrogen from the protein carrier in the blood. DHA increases estrogen levels and can increase aromatase enzymes[221]. Aromatase enzymes can convert testosterone into estrogen. The decrease in temperature increase estrogen receptors and an increase in temperature decreases its affinity (more estrogen may be required for a response)[222]. The addition of thyroid reduces estrogen receptors, while hypothyroid organisms up-regulate the estrogen receptor. The thyroid up-regulates the androgen receptor, possibly increasing their affinity[223].

Furthermore, DHA and EPA can decrease the androgen receptors and can inhibit the 5alpha reductase (5-DHT) enzyme. Thyroid and caffeine (heat-increasing molecules) increase 5alpha reductase activity and decrease desaturase enzymes that omega-3 and omega-6 use[224][225]. The unsaturated fats selectively inhibit the 5-alpha reductase enzymes, while saturated fats were found to be inactive[226]. A simple description of the aromatase enzyme is seen below.

Fish oil can decrease the androgen receptors and can inhibit the 5alpha reductase (5-DHT) enzyme

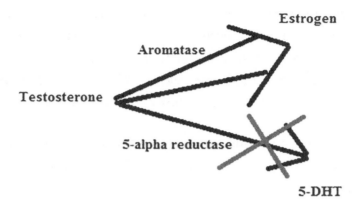

As fish oils can activate genes to decrease cholesterol production, they also affect the enzymes that contribute to a healthy steroid profile. The conversion of the parent hormone pregnenolone into the other hormone depends on specific enzymes. Fish oil is known to down-regulate these enzymes leading to decreasing the supply to the next hormone. Fish oil is known to down-regulate P450c17 that converts pregnenolone to DHEA and hydroxysteroid sulfotransferase (SULT) that turns DHEA into DHEA-S, all of which have health attributes and decline during aging[227].

DHT "Toxic Masculinity"

"Further, epidemiologic studies indicate that elevated estrogen levels in utero can predispose to an increased risk of prostate cancer later in life"[228]

Calderon-Gierszal EL, Prins GS (2015) Directed Differentiation of Human Embryonic Stem Cells into Prostate Organoids In Vitro and its Perturbation by Low-Dose Bisphenol A Exposure. PLoS ONE 10 (7): e0133238. https://doi.org/10.1371/journal.pone.0133238

"Early estrogen exposure alone affects branching morphogenesis, leading to the presence of rudimentary glands, and hinders basal cell communication. These estrogenic effects are persistent and present in a 200-day differentiated adult gland"[229]

Saffarini CM, McDonnell-Clark EV, Amin A, Huse SM, Boekelheide K (2015) Developmental Exposure to Estrogen Alters Differentiation and Epigenetic Programming in a Human Fetal Prostate Xenograft Model. PLoS ONE 10 (3): e0122290. https://doi.org/10.1371/journal.pone.0122290

Although 5-DHT is demonized and blamed for many illnesses, at normal psychological levels, this hormone is quite healthy as it may have cognitive-enhancing properties[230][231]. A reduction in 5-DHT often translates into a reduction in male fertility health. 5-DHT is seen as one of the primary hormones for healthy bones, muscles, and strength. The lowering of 5-DHT due to omega-3 by blocking 5-alpha-reductase leaves the omega-3 brain-boosting properties less likely (besides lowering omega-6).

Recently, studies have shown that testosterone and 5-DHT might not be the culprit in prostate difficulties and could be part of a solution[232][233] (low DHT is associated with higher mortality from prostate cancer[234]). It has been shown that DHT is very neuroprotective (reduced thiobarbituric acid-reactive substance levels and improved mitochondria), which is linked to DHT and not its metabolites. Fish oils are positively associated with prostate cancer[235][236]. *In 1993, it was demonstrated that although the 5-DHT can be increased in human benign prostatic hyperplasia (especially epithelium), they also showed a "dramatic" increase in estrogen in the stroma compared to 5-DHT[237]. This altered ratio in favor of estrogen disturbs the synergism between the androgen-estrogen balance needed to produce and maintain a healthy prostate[238], especially in childhood[239]. This accumulation of estrogen was demonstrated in 1982[240]. The limited success in BHP with 5-alpha-reductase can easily be contributed to lower estrogen levels as DHT can convert into molecules with estrogenic properties[241] without the use of aromatase.*

Progesterone And Fish Oil

As progesterone declines during aging, lipid peroxidation increases. The same seems to correlate well with DHEA: as we age, there is a decline with DHEA and a subsequent rise in MDA (fish oil breakdown product)[242]. In women, low estradiol blood levels (below 50 pg/ml) and, more dangerously, above 299 pg/ml were found to see an increase in lipid peroxidation[243]. 'Normal' levels are seen as between 50-400. At the different periods of ovulation, progesterone levels can be 100 times as high to offer protection. It has been found that low basal body temperature (too little progesterone, excess estrogen) is a reason for miscarriage[244] or difficulties getting pregnant. Progesterone should not be confused with progestins (synthetic progesterone). Progesterone is a heat-producing hormone and is dose-dependent inhibited by fish oils[245][246]. Fish oils change the ratio between progesterone and estrogen.

Soy Boy

"The increase in obesity in the U.S. over the last half-century coincides with a shift in the dietary preference away from saturated fats from animal products and toward plant-based unsaturated fats"[247]

Deol P, Evans JR, Dhahbi J, Chellappa K, Han DS, Spindler S, et al. (2015) Soybean Oil Is More Obesogenic and Diabetogenic than Coconut Oil and Fructose in Mouse: Potential Role for the Liver. PLoS ONE 10 (7): e0132672. https://doi.org/10.1371/journal.pone.0132672

Soy has one of the highest amounts of (omega-3) alpha-linolenic acid in foods, as in ocean-based organisms, soy increases its unsaturated fatty acid content at lower temperatures[248]. As the unsaturated fats increase in cold weather, so does the estrogen content. The well-known phytoestrogens genistein and daidzein have estrogen activity and are well-known infertility ingredients. It is interesting to note that cold weather induces an increase in these ingredients[249]. This is in line with the formation of unsaturated fats in cold weather and saturated fats in warm weather. Both males and females are affected by soy: in men, it lowers sperm count and reduced mobility[250]; in women, it can increase the possibility of miscarriage and reduces the rate of offspring[251]. Both soy and estrogen can increase cortisol[252][253]. In the USA, soy oil intake saw an 1163-fold increase from 1900-2000[254]. The two most significant increases in obesity in the US correspond well with the rise of soy oil around 1970 and canola oil around 1988. It is my opinion that soy-oil, together with the other PUFA, is partly responsible for the decrease of manhood (testosterone[255], DHT[256][257], and strength) seen in the Western world during this and the previous century.

Desaturase Enzymes Are Disastrous

"These results identify D6D as a key factor for tumor growth and as a potential target for cancer therapy and prevention"[258]

He C, Qu X, Wan J, Rong R, Huang L, Cai C, et al. (2012) Inhibiting Delta-6 Desaturase Activity Suppresses Tumor Growth in Mice. PLoS ONE 7 (10): e47567. https://doi.org/10.1371/journal.pone.0047567

Delta-6-desaturase (D6D) and delta-5-desaturase (D5D) enzymes are seen as crucial for health as they are capable of converting the essential fatty acids from the parents' fats. Both linolenic acid and linoleic acids need these enzymes to create more double bonds and elongate the carbon chain. What is not often mentioned is the fact that these enzymes are associated with a host of potential problems. The previously mentioned D-6-D can be followed by enzyme D-5-D (and D-4-D) for the conversion into DHA. When the DNA codes for D-5-D are deleted in mice, the effects are dramatic. These D-5-D absent mice are leaner, more active, have better glucose and insulin levels, and show up to a 40% reduction in atherosclerosis (cholesterol levels were similar, indicating that cholesterol is not the main culprit in atherosclerosis)[259]. Another study found that a D-5-D inhibitor resulted in increased insulin sensitivity, increased weight loss, and increased energy expenditure[260], both levels of omega-3 and omega-6 AA and EPA/DHA levels decreased dramatically. To the scientists' surprise, there was no abnormality associated with the inhibition of these enzymes and a decrease of the longer unsaturated fats.

Troglitazone, used for diabetes, is a known D-5-D reducer[261]. Delta-6-desaturase inhibition has been shown to reverse cardiolipin remodeling, (which occurs when DHA and long-chain omega-6 fatty acids accumulate). It prevents contractile dysfunction in the aged mouse heart[262].

EPA can reduce D-5-D and D-6-D that leads to reduced arachidonic acid blood content by downregulating de desaturase enzymes. Again, this positive quality of EPA can also be achieved by limiting AA (or other omega-6) in the first place. The unsaturated fats themselves also act as a negative feedback loop. When unsaturated fats are consumed, the enzymes that make unsaturated fats more unsaturated are reduced[263]. *D-5-D has an inverse relation with the active thyroid hormone T3, as D-5-D goes up in hunger, hibernation, limited resources, T3 goes down[264], and the addition of T3 decreases D-5-D and D-6-D[265].*

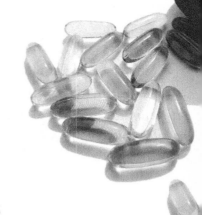

CHAPTER 4

Health Of The Fatty Fish Eaters

N atives in the Arctic have had high mortality from infections in the past and still do today. Recently, it was discovered that the aforementioned FADS-1 gene has an unhealthy relationship with tuberculosis. This gene can increase the omega-6 to omega-3 ratio of 26 to 1 to about 3 to 1. When this gene was inserted into mice, they showed an increase in susceptibility to tuberculosis (TB) and a decrease in resistance to the infection. The scientists warned to investigate and be cautious with omega-3 supplementation in areas with high tuberculosis risk[266].

"However, our findings raise questions regarding the safety of n-3 supplementation. An improved understanding of the lipid effect on intracellular infections, including TB, will allow a better assessment of the potential health risks of excessive intake of n-3 PUFA in humans, leading to the establishment of dietary guidelines to avoid detrimental effects. We hypothesize that diets supplemented with n-3 PUFA increase host susceptibility to TB infection in vivo."[267]

Bonilla DL, Ly LH, Fan Y-Y, Chapkin RS, McMurray DN (2010) Incorporation of a Dietary Omega 3 Fatty Acid Impairs Murine Macrophage Responses to Mycobacterium tuberculosis. PLoS ONE 5 (5): e10878. https://doi.org/10.1371/journal.pone.0010878

Natives From The North

Many of the natives around the Arctic have been viewed as a picture of perfect health living off the land and sea. The view of the Arctic natives has contributed to the popularity of the ketogenic-like diets. The alleged absence of enough carbohydrates in the Arctic combined with the ideas of 'athletic' natives can be traced back centuries. From many investigatory accounts, we can see that these natives were almost never in a severe ketogenic state. Natives often ate tissues rich in glycogen and lean meat, which can be transformed into sugars. At the northern Arctic, fish was not eaten that often, while seal and walrus, narwhal, and hare were commonly consumed. As the weather became warmer, the fat intake of the natives could be as low as about 15%[268]. The natives often ate whale and the whole fish. Whale contains high amounts of vitamin E (more than five times as much as sardine). Vitamin E is protective against some of the (side) effects of EPA/DHA.

Native populations often ate more seal and lean meat than fish, which contains less polyunsaturated fats (PUFA)[269]. Furthermore, natives from near the Arctic seem to have a different constitution. This constitution keeps their arachidonic acid (omega-6) low, even on a Western diet (the desaturase enzymes work differently), leading to lower AA even in a low EPA environment[270].

Natives Elsewhere

This book will not go in-depth on this topic, but observations and studies are indicating that some of the tribes in the Arctic had a good standard of health. To attribute good health solely to the fats in the diet seems less logical when comparing the health of the tribes living on little or no essential fats. The aforementioned Maasai ate little omega-3 while enjoying a high level of health. Furthermore, well-nourished peoples from the West Indies in Indonesia lived on about 20 grams of total fat per day, which were mostly saturated fats. During World War II, areas of occupied Holland experienced famine for months during the last year of the war. Hundreds of thousands of people averaged about 4 grams of fat per day for months. After the liberation, apart from vitamin deficiencies and starvation, no signs were found that could be attributed to the absence of essential fatty acids[271].

Fodor and colleagues in 2014 shook the scientific community by reviewing the evidence of fatty fish intake and Coronary artery disease (CAD). Fodor showed that the diet of the Greenland Natives and the low CAD was not supported by substantial evidence[272]. I would like to go into some additional studies and reviews to support the notion that native fish-eating populations were not as healthy as often portrayed.

Native Cold Fish-Eating Populations And Health

In 1913, a medical doctor named Watkins, onboard the U.S.S Bear, visited and rendered aid to different villages along the Alaskan coast. Of the 281 cases reviewed, they encountered a high percentage of eye problems (33%)[273]. In 1935, a team of researchers went to the Canadian Arctic to investigate the condition and health of

Canadian natives. The lead researcher, Rabinowitch, was interested in the alleged absence of arteriosclerosis and other diseases. Rabinowitch, in his investigation, collected x-ray data from the natives and found that the percentage of atherosclerosis was in line with the national average. He concluded that his evidence proved that the alleged absence of heart problems had been disproven in the eastern Arctic[274].

Several institutions, like the Norwegian Polar Institute, surveyed and summarized the following observations regarding health and disease amongst the natives.

- The father of Greenland epidemiology - Bertelson - commented that arteriosclerosis and an aging myocardium are common among the Inuit[275].
- Hoygaard, who studied natives in the southeast of Greenland in 1941, mentioned that arteriosclerosis was often found in people under age 40[276].
- Brown argued that the low cancer rate could be because of the young age of the natives and provided examples of atherosclerosis in these people[277].
- Further studies regarding natives continued into the 1950s that showed that cholesterol serum was at about the same levels as white people[278].
- In 1960, Gottman found that in autopsied natives from Alaska, atherosclerotic cardiovascular disease was not uncommon[279]. While two years later, Lederman concluded after the autopsy of 90 Alaskan natives that Eskimos do have atherosclerosis[280].

- Around the same time, the incidence of arthritis in the natives' population was found to be the same as white people[281].
- They found cancer to be common in the native population in southwest Alaska, despite contrary beliefs in 1969[282].
- In 1974, it was observed that the bone loss of the Alaskan natives occurred more aggressively and at an earlier age[283].
- Alaskan Eskimos were found to have average cholesterol of 214.4 mg per 100 ml and slightly higher blood pressure than the US average[284].
- The Natives of Canada (Northwest passage) were found to have normal cholesterol levels 160-250 mg/dl, which increased with aging[285].

These and other studies accumulated into a paper by the Division for Research in Greenland, National Institute of Public Health in 2002. The document states that mortality of stroke is the same or even higher within the Inuit community, compared to the westerners. Furthermore, the evidence for low death from Ischemic Heart Disease (IHD) is unreliable[286].

Natives Nowadays

When comparing Omega-3 intakes of the different regions in Alaska, one can find some interesting associations. The areas of Alaska with a higher omega-3 intake show the highest heart disease mortality compared to areas with lower consumption. Both the Interior (lowest with 138.6 per 100,000) and Southeast (third lowest with 147.9 per 100,000) have a significantly lower intake of omega-3 compared to the Yukon-Kuskokwim (273.7 per 100,000) which had high (er) amounts of omega-3 intakes. Interior and Southeast regions also show lower deaths from cancer than

Yukon-Kuskokwim[287288]. The Alaskan Eskimos consuming vast quantities of omega-3 versus those having fewer amounts showed no difference with regards to Coronary Heart Disease (CHD). One study showed that Eskimos classified as CHD had non-significant higher levels of omega-3 serum levels and intake[289].

HsCRP (High-sensitivity C-reactive protein) is a marker for many pathologies ranging from heart disease to cancer. Another protein (Glyco) that is a marker is called YKL-40. In 2013, it was revealed that as Inuit were consuming a more traditional diet, markers of atherosclerosis and inflammation (YKL-40 and hsCRP) were high both compared with non-Inuit and with Inuit that was consuming a non-traditional diet[290]. Omega-3 intake was not associated with reduced carotid atherosclerosis among Alaska natives[291]. The average consumption by Alaskan native men was between 5.9 grams and 4.9 grams per day. These Alaskan Eskimo had higher rates of carotid atherosclerosis, but smoking could be a cause[292]. Compared to the Danish Caucasian population, Greenland natives have three times an increased chance of bleeding intracranial aneurysms[293].

But Cold Fish-Eating Countries Are Healthier, Surely?

Many articles make the association between the fish oil intake (in the form of fish, not supplements) and low prevalence of heart disease. The most common countries to focus upon are Iceland, Norway, and Japan. While seafood consumption and, therefore, fish oil consumption is higher in those countries (together with minerals and other useful molecules), the levels of omega-6 intake in those same countries are among the lowest. *Countries that consume low amounts of omega-3 (fish and seafood) like Luxembourg[294], the Swiss, Israel, and Ireland[295] have comparable numbers regarding heart disease[296297]. In Europe, the countries with the highest PUFA intake have the highest heart disease mortality.*

In the 1990s, health organizations advised that no more than 7% of total energy intake should come from PUFA[298]. The current recommendations are 6-11% of energy from PUFA[299]. European countries that have high PUFA intakes like Russia, Bulgaria, and Hungary, but medium or even low saturated fat[300] intake had the highest rate of cardiovascular disease[301].

Japan

The Japanese have spent a lot of time researching fish oil. They found that fish oils were not that toxic as long as they were stable and did not come in contact with oxygen and other compounds. The oxygenation of these oils caused rapid lipid peroxidation.

Although touted as having an omega-3 loaded diet, research shows that the fish intake in Japan since 1950 has stayed relatively the same, while eggs, meat, and fruit intake increased. The decline in cancer rates is positively correlated with the most significant increase in meat, eggs, and fruit intake, not fish intake[302]. Recently it was shown that coronary heart disease declined in Japan between 1980-2008, "despite" rising cholesterol levels[303]. Japan has an overall low iron intake, and its diet has a high amount of iron inhibitors (green tea, and specific ingredients in soy[304305]).

One of the longest-living peoples has, until recently, been the people of Okinawa. Their traditional diet comprised high carbohydrate (mostly sweet potato), low protein, and low-fat levels of 6%. The traditional food of Okinawa was compared to the Japanese menu. It was found that the Okinawa diet was lower in calories and more plentiful in minerals and vitamins (especially vitamin A, potassium, and vitamin E). The fish intake was about 1/4 of the rest of Japan at the same time (1949-1950)[306]. Data from Japan during 1980-1999 showed that eating fish more than twice per week had no benefit compared to twice a week fish consumption concerning total mortality[307]. *Quantities of peroxides in the blood follow the amount of omega-3 intakes. When the Japanese are compared to Americans and Japanese living in the USA, it can be seen that the Japanese have the highest amount of omega-3 in the blood, followed by Japanese residing in the USA, while Americans had the lowest (omega-6 was lowest in those living in Japan). Also, the Japanese had the highest TBAR, followed by Japanese in the USA and lowest in Americans[308].*

Norway

"Fish, and particularly lean fish, is a major part of the Norwegian diet, especially for people living along the Norwegian coastline"[309]

Rylander C, Sandanger TM, Engeset D, Lund E (2014) Consumption of Lean Fish Reduces the Risk of Type 2 Diabetes Mellitus: A Prospective Population Based Cohort Study of Norwegian Women. PLoS ONE 9 (2): e89845. https://doi.org/10.1371/journal.pone.0089845

As it is surrounded by different seas, Norway's consumption of fish is among the highest in the world and is often mentioned regarding health. Headlines range from how a Nordic diet can decrease the chances of getting cancer and/or diabetes and should be adopted by other countries, according to the World Health Organization. Norway, in its current state, is among the lowest heart disease countries. However, 30 years ago, Norway and Denmark were noted to oppose the fish-eating hypothesis that a high fish diet contributes to moderate levels of heart disease.

"Clearly by careful selection of countries, for example contrasting Switzerland and Yugoslavia (low fish and low CHD) with Denmark and Norway (high fish and moderately high CHD) one could propose that fish caused rather than prevented CHD" [310]

Reproduced from 37 Words (p. 563). I. K. Crombie et al. International differences in coronary heart disease mortality and consumption of fish and other foodstuffs. European Heart Journal (1987) 8 (6): 560-563, doi: 10.1093/oxfordjournals.eurheartj.a062322. By permission of Oxford University Press on behalf of the ESC.

The neighboring country of Norway is Sweden, which is not often mentioned. Norway's omega-3 intake is almost double that of Sweden. When looking at heart disease, Sweden has lower numbers than Norway regarding mortality in stroke, CHD, CVD, and total numbers. Again, reinforcing the message that more fish oil is likely not better (Sweden consumes more saturated fats than Norway)[311]. In Norway, higher DHA levels in membranes are associated with postoperative atrial fibrillation[312].

Iceland

Iceland probably has the highest intake of seafood per person[313]. In the 1990s, Iceland was known for having a high fish intake and a high coronary heart disease (CHD) incidence. Iceland has been in the news as it has seen a massive decline in heart disease from 1981 to 2006. It was calculated that the almost 75% decrease of CHD deaths was attributed to lifestyle changes. Within this time, among other factors, fish consumption had come down from 73 grams per day in 1990 to 27 grams in 2004[314]. In 2011, research in Iceland found that higher levels of DHA in the heart of pre and post-operative stages found increase postoperative atrial fibrillation (POAF), the higher levels of DHA, the higher incidence of POAF was found[315].

CHAPTER 5

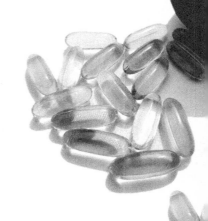

| Unsaturated Fat, Fragile Fat

| Lipid Peroxidation: Initiation, Propagation, Termination, Initiation, Propagation, Termination, Initiation…

"As the most sensitive chemical functional groups in biological molecules, unsaturated fatty acids essentially harvest oxidizing potential from the atmosphere and transform it into highly reactive chemical species"[316]

Schaich, K.M. 2014. Lipid co-oxidation of proteins: One size does not fit all. Inform, 25 (3): 134-139.

Apart from fish oils (and other PUFA) in their complete form, there is something else that makes fish oil not suitable for their isolated intake. The presence of double bonds in unsaturated fats makes these molecules prone to peroxidation. This peroxidation is not the burning of fat for energy, which is known as beta-oxidation. Lipid peroxidation is the degradation of fats initiated by free radicals.

How Does It Happen?

The presence of double bonds changes the configuration of hydrogen bonds compared to saturated fats. This configuration weakens the linkage between the hydrogen atom and the carbon atom next to the double bond (allylic hydrogens). When carbons are surrounded by double bonds (on each side), it is even more loosely attached (bis-allylic). EPA has 4 bis-allylic methyl groups, while DHA has 5.

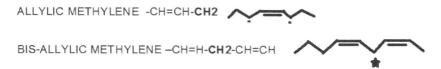

ALLYLIC METHYLENE -CH=CH-**CH2**

BIS-ALLYLIC METHYLENE –CH=H-**CH2**-CH=CH

Dots denote allytic; Star denote Bis-allylic

As was mentioned in previous chapters, fats comprise of a carbon backbone surrounded by hydrogen atoms. These hydrogen atoms are more loosely connected with polyunsaturated fats than with saturated or mono-unsaturated fats. Hydrogen is the smallest and lightest element and can be abstracted easily. Scientists can add a neutron to hydrogen (deuterated hydrogen) to make it heavier and more resistant from becoming dislodged. When protium hydrogen (without a neutron) is replaced with deuterated hydrogen and given to organisms, lifespans are increased compared to organisms with normal hydrogen[317]. Free radicals can take the loosened hydrogen, and this is known as a hydrogen abstraction (hydrogen steal). This action makes the radical stable, but, makes the lipid molecule unstable and is known as the initiation of lipid peroxidation. Oxygen can attach itself to the unstable lipid creating a peroxyl radical (LOO*). LOO* looks for another hydrogen to steal, from another unsaturated acid (propagation). This, in turn, will create a lipid peroxide (LOOH) ending the lipid peroxidation process (termination) for this unsaturated fat, while starting another peroxyl radical. This cycle can go on and on and on.

The whole process of lipid peroxidation occurs in 3 stages. On the following page, the three stages of lipid peroxidation are shown. These three stages are initiation, propagation, and termination.

See the description on the next page of the 3 stages (adapted from Elinder F and Liin SI (2017) Actions and Mechanisms of Polyunsaturated Fatty Acids on Voltage-Gated Ion Channels. Front. Physiol. 8:43. doi: 10.3389/fphys.2017.00043).

Lipid peroxidation

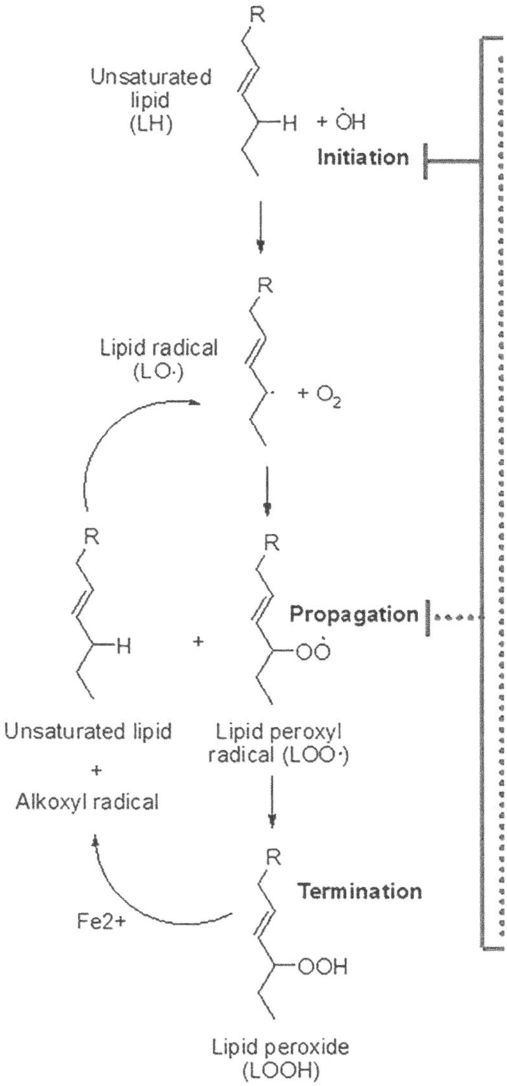

R
Unsaturated lipid (LH)
H + ȮH
Initiation
R
Lipid radical (LO·)
+ O_2
R
R
Propagation
H
+
OȮ
Unsaturated lipid
+
Alkoxyl radical
Lipid peroxyl radical (LOȮ·)
R
Termination
Fe2+
OOH
Lipid peroxide (LOOH)

Initiation

The loosening of the bond between hydrogen and carbon because of the double carbon bond is an easy target for free radicals. This hydrogen atom is up for grabs for unstable molecules (radicals). DHA has 5 bis-allylic methylene groups that can be easily abstracted. To compare this with monounsaturated fat that has no bis-allylic methylene group, DHA is according to some accounts 320 times more susceptible to be attacked and eight times more likely than 18:2n-6. Furthermore, fish oils can be broken down into many different dangerous molecules[318]. Although lipid peroxidation needs a free radical to start, once the initiation has begun, it becomes autocatalytic (self-propagating and also self-accelerating). The initiation can occur quickly in any of the natural states of lipids.

These include:

- Triacylglycerols (fatty acids as stored as triacylglycerols).
- Free fatty acids, after fatty acids are released from phospholipids or triacylglycerols.
- Phospholipids - lipids are part of phospholipids, usually as part of cell membranes.
- Fatty acids can be attached to other molecules like transporting proteins (known as waxes).

The abstraction of the hydrogen molecule from the unsaturated fatty acid leaves the carbon molecule unpaired and means it can become a radical. Hydroxyl radical seems to be the most frequent initiator of lipid peroxidation. It has been estimated that every second, 50 hydroxyl radicals can be generated in one cell. This radical causes rearrangement of double bonds, creating conjugated dienes to become peroxyl radical after combining with oxygen. The peroxyl radical can perpetuate the wave of events by attacking other polyunsaturated fats. Below is a quick description of initiation and propagation.

Propagation

The real damage occurs during the propagation phase. The propagation phase is the second part of lipid peroxidation and is also known as the branching phase. The radical from the initiation phase comes in contact with oxygen. This action changes L into LOO*, which are known as reactive peroxyl radicals. These reactive peroxyl radicals are unstable and take hydrogen from other lipids to form hydroperoxides: LOOH (lipid peroxide). This action leads into a new series of forming L radicals that abstract hydrogen atoms until there are no more hydrogens to take or anti-oxidants to stop the reaction.

Termination

The phrase termination means that the initiation molecule is stopped from being a radical. This change from radical to nonradical can occur in various forms: radical recombination, alpha and beta scission reactions of alkoxyl radicals, co-oxidation with proteins, group eliminations, or dismutation. It is important to note that although the initial lipid is stopped from being a radical, the other fats affected can continue the process[319]. Also notable is the fact that damage has already occurred - co-oxidation with proteins, for example, can make the protein less functional. Fish oil can be degraded into numerous compounds that consist of alkenes, aldehydes, ketones, epoxides, and many more volatile products[320].

How Fish Oil Can Decrease Inflammation

Inflammation (after lipid peroxidation) up-regulates enzymes like catalase and glutathione peroxidase and superoxide dismutase. Some argue that a small degree of lipid oxidation is a healthy way to upregulate anti-inflammatory response, resulting in better health. This might be true in limited amounts, but not necessary for the fish oil, which breaks down products that could include acrolein, aldehydes, and lipofuscin. Furthermore, too much inflammation can result in a state in which the anti-inflammatory enzymes are used up and cannot be recycled fast enough or are unable to perform their actions (by lipofuscin for example). These enzymes are unable to perform at their regular rates and reactive oxygen species, and most likely, aging is sped up. One way by which fish oils can decrease inflammation is by the Keap1–Nrf2–ARE Pathway.

The breakdown products of fish oil can activate anti-inflammatory genes leading to anti-inflammatory enzymes like (GSH, HO-1). DHA can break down in 4-HHE, 4-HHE, in turn, can steal an electron from the KEAP-1-Nrf2 molecule, Nrf2 can get detached from KEAP-1 and go from the cytosol into the nucleus for gene transcription instead of being identified for degradation. Nrf2 goes into the nucleus and activate Antioxidant Response Element (ARE) molecules, which have anti-inflammatory activities (see picture below).

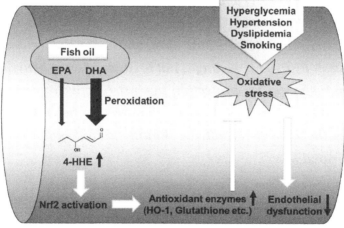

Aortic tissue

From: Ishikado A, Morino K, Nishio Y, Nakagawa F, Mukose A, Sono Y, et al. (2013) 4-Hydroxy Hexenal Derived from Docosahexaenoic Acid Protects Endothelial Cells via Nrf2 Activation. PLoS ONE 8 (7): e69415. https://doi. org/10.1371/journal.pone.0069415

The science about Nrf2 is not settled, as Nrf2 can be overexpressed in cancers[321]. Furthermore, in brain diseases like Alzheimer's and Parkinson's disease, the problem is not a lack of Nrf2, but rather the difficulties of Nrf2 getting into the nucleus of the cell, making high levels Nnrf2 not necessarily very helpful[322].

To associate fish oil with health because of its increase in Nrf2 makes less sense as known poisons like methyl mercury makes cells behave the same way. In this line of thinking, methylmercury could be considered a health supplement[323]! In animals were Nrf2 are positively associated with longevity, it also shows a negative association with keap1[324]. Chronically elevated levels of Nrf2 can be detrimental to longevity[325].

Instead of fish oil supplementation, exercise can activate Nrf2 levels and even can achieve the same positive effects independent of Nrf2. At the same time, exercise can decrease 4-HNE accumulation[326]. This upregulation of antioxidant gene expression by fish oil feeding is not because of some benefit to the human body, but for protection against reactive oxygen species produced by fish oil[327]. It has been known that fish oil is prone to damage the tissue and challenge the antioxidant system compared to saturated fats[328].

"The accumulation of high levels of the toxic lipid oxidation product 4-HHE may endanger microglia"[329]

Yip, Ping & Pizzasegola, Chiara & Gladman, Stacy & Biggio, Maria & Marino, Marianna & Jayasinghe, Maduka & Ullah, Farhan & Dyall, Simon & Malaspina, Andrea & Bendotti, Caterina & Michael-Titus, Adina. (2013). The Omega-3 Fatty Acid Eicosapentaenoic Acid Accelerates Disease Progression in a Model of Amyotrophic Lateral Sclerosis. PloS one. 8. e61626. 10.1371/journal.pone.0061626.

Testing and Results

"The most challenging aspect of studying ROS metabolism is the fact that they are extremely reactive and short-lived molecules, which make them difficult to measure. Various approaches have been developed for cell-based systems to measure ROS and ROS damage, but many suffer from a lack of specificity, linearity or detailed method characterization"[330]

Labuschagne CF, van den Broek NJF, Postma P, Berger R, Brenkman AB (2013) A Protocol for Quantifying Lipid Peroxidation in Cellular Systems by F2-Isoprostane Analysis. PLoS ONE 8 (11): e80935. https://doi.org/10.1371/journal.pone.0080935

Already in 1961, research showed that fish oil could break down in at least 28 carbonyls and many unknown compounds[331]. A couple of years later, methanol and propanal were detected[332]. In 2005, over 200 gaseous products had been found. The problem is that only about 10% of the total known products seem to have any relation to the sensory test used[333]. Until today the best way of testing for the rancidity of fish oil is for experienced humans to do sensory (taste panels) tests. Humans can detect meager amounts of volatile products better than other ways of mechanical testing. This way of testing is problematic, as most people are not keen to take part in this kind of testing. Studies with grants from toxicity research departments, published in the Journal of Food Technologies, showed that auto-oxidized fish oils contained alkenes, malondialdehyde, ketones, monocarbonyls, and many additional compounds that could not be identified[334][335]. The Journal of Food Technologies has published these studies for 50-plus years, without permeating to popular magazines[336]. In the following table, some of the more popular ways of testing are described, as well as their potential problems.

Some of the most common testing methods are described on the next page, as well as the problems associated with them.

Test	Measurement	Problem
Color	A dark color may be reflected of rancidity and or contaminants	No standard
Peroxide values (PV)	Measurement of primary products	It only measures primary products.
P-anisidine number (AN),	Measures peroxide levels	Only oxidation numbers from the past, no standard
TOTOX numbers	A combination of 2 * PV + AN	It only measures the current state, not for future measurement
Iodine value (IV)	High IV indicates higher unsaturation	No standard
Acid Value	Measures the acid value, high acid crude fish oil levels indicate poor quality fish oil	No longer used
Moisture	Moisture can lead to deterioration in storage	Only test up to date, does not predict oxidation levels
Impurity test	This test can measure elements that can be pro-oxidant (iron, copper, lead, arsenic, selenium, cadmium, mercury)	Usually no standard
Thiobarbituric (TBA) value	A method that rate aldehyde products	Is not specific and limited (aldehydes)

Most testing for lipid peroxidation measures the hydroperoxidation after initiation during propagation. Hydroperoxidation is the initial oxidative product that is formed, and this is one of the tests that GOED recommends for testing fish oils. The problem with this measurement is the fact that fish oil can be oxidized into secondary volatile products so quickly. The GOED and most independent testing for secondary products are based on adisine values. Adisine values test the aldehydes and TOTOX, which test both hydroperoxides and adisine together[337].

Research Of Fish Oil Versus Vegetable Oil

One problem with fish oils is the immaturity of its research. While much of the analysis of vegetable oil started in the 1970s, fish oil research is still in its infancy and only really began in the mid-1990s. Looking at the PubMed database, there is a clear difference in focus when studying different fats. This focus is logical because there is more consumption of omega-6 than omega-3, but this focus plays into the view that fish oil is not that bad. The terms "health" and DHA and EPA yield more research articles than AA articles. At the same time, "lipid peroxidation" generates fewer items with DHA and EPA than AA. This can mean that the focus is on the combination of DHA, EPA, and health, not on lipid peroxidation. Luckily, the research is catching up, as is shown in the figure comparing fatty acids and lipid peroxidation.

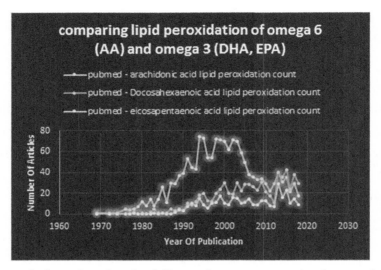

The graph above describes the difference between omega-6 and omega-3 and "lipid peroxidation" using the PubMed database. The left axis (Y-axis) shows the number of articles. The bottom axis (X-axis) displays the year of publication. Especially during the 1980s, 1990s, and 2000s, the omega-6 fats were heavily researched (more so than now), while the omega-3 only recently saw an increase.

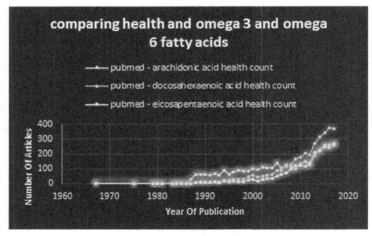

The graph above describes the difference between omega-6 and omega-3 and "health" using the PubMed database. The left axis (Y-axis) shows the number of articles. The bottom axis (X-axis) displays the year of publication. While the research on omega-6 has remained largely constant, the omega-3 research in combination with health has exploded since the 2000s.

Fish Oil: Some Molecules to Mention

"Particularly damaging, ROS can initiate a free radical chain-reaction in unsaturated fatty acids, thereby generating toxic electrophilic α/β unsaturated aldehydes, a process called lipid peroxidation. The best characterized of these carbonyl-derivatives are 4-hydroxy-2-nonenal (4-HNE), malondialdehyde (MDA) and acrolein"[338]

Petersen DR, Saba LM, Sayin VI, Papagiannakopoulos T, Schmidt EE, Merrill GF, et al. (2018) Elevated Nrf-2 responses are insufficient to mitigate protein carbonylation in hepatospecific PTEN deletion mice. PLoS ONE 13 (5): e0198139. https://doi.org/10.1371/journal.pone.0198139

Fish oil can form through non-enzymatic peroxidation into many molecules. Although much data is missing and are yet to be elucidated, some pathways are described. As is mentioned in the quote above, 4-HNE, MDA, and acrolein are most well known, but there are many others. In the following paragraphs, some of these molecules are described, and their effects are noted. Important to note is that 4-HNE can be derived from omega-6. 4-HNE has an isomer that can be derived from omega-3. This isomer is called Trans-4-Hydroxy-2-Hexenal (HHE). HHE escapes most of the research, as the focus is on HNE. Isomers are molecules that have similar amounts of atoms, but some molecules are in different places.

Trans-4-Hydroxy-2-Hexenal (HHE)

"In line with this matter, increased levels of LCPUFA–derived lipid hydroperoxides like HHE, HNE, and other endoperoxides like isoprostanes have been observed in the brain of transgenic models of Alzheimer's disease"[339]

Casañas-Sánchez V, Pérez JA, Fabelo N, Quinto-Alemany D and Díaz ML (2015) Docosahexaenoic (DHA) modulates phospholipid-hydroperoxide glutathione peroxidase (Gpx4) gene expression to ensure self-protection from oxidative damage in hippocampal cells. Front. Physiol. 6:203. doi: 10.3389/fphys.2015.00203

One of the breakdown products of fish oil is the before mentioned trans-4-hydroxy-2-hexenal (HHE). HHE is the isomer of the omega-6 vegetable oil HNE. HNE (omega-6) was found to be toxic in the late 1970s and causes an overall decrease in energy[340]. Only around 1985 was it discovered that trans-4-hydroxy-2-hexenal (HHE) was a breakdown product of DHA[341]. HHE is involved in an increase in DNA damage, protein and phospholipid adducts, cytotoxicity and apoptosis, and a decrease in GSH (anti-inflammatory enzyme).

How Does It Work?

Because of the fragile attachment of the hydrogen to the unsaturated fats, fragments of fats can be created. Displayed below is how HHE is formed from DHA:

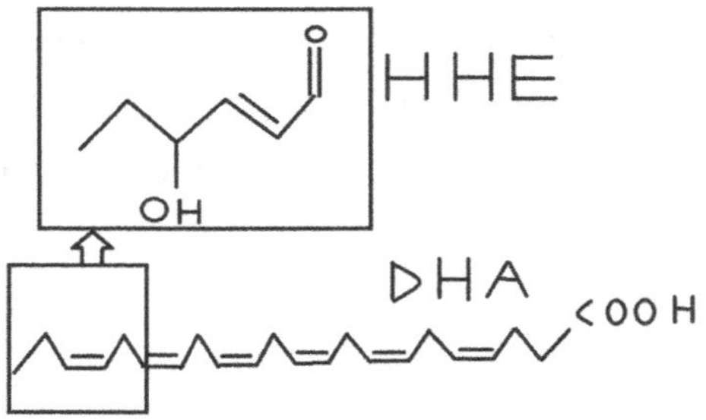

Like many other breakdown products of fish oil, HHE is found in the initial stages of plaque formation (foam cells). HHE can be incorporated into macrophages and change the proteins in such a way that they cannot be broken down by enzymes and get stuck in the arteries forming foam cells. Furthermore, LDL particles with HHE can create oxidized LDL, leading to the uptake of these dangerous LDL particles into cells, thus leading to the accumulation of plaque[342]. The graph below illustrates the difference between HHE and HNE research, even though they have many of the same adverse effects.

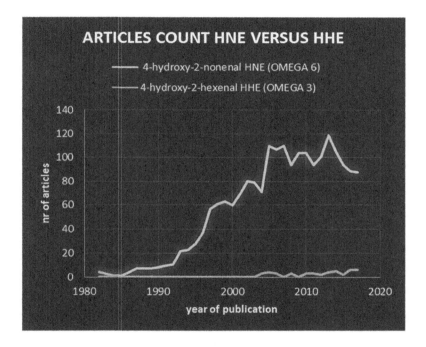

Malondialdehyde

"Malondialdehyde (MDA) is widely used as a marker for the peroxidation of ω 3 and ω 6 fatty acids."[343]

Kapusta A, Kuczyńska B, Puppel K (2018) Relationship between the degree of antioxidant protection and the level of malondialdehyde in high-performance Polish Holstein-Friesian cows in peak of lactation. PLoS ONE 13 (3): e0193512. https://doi.org/10.1371/journal.pone.0193512

Malondialdehyde can be increased by supplementing with fish oil[344345346347348]. The creation of malondialdehyde is exceptionally high in the second part of the small intestine (duodenal), making blood testing unreliable. Malondialdehyde is also used as a marker as oxidative status [349] and possibly aging[350]. Furthermore, malondialdehyde formation can be seen as a deficiency in antioxidant systems. On the next page is a depiction of how lysine and malondialdehyde can interact, causing lysine to be less functional.

Malondialdehyde can link up with lysine and make lysine less functional. Malondialdehyde attached to lysine is found in many pathologies. Malondialdehyde can link up with many amino acids.

"MDA modifies the physical structures of cell membranes and is indirectly involved in the synthesis of protein, DNA, and RNA. In addition, it has mutagenic and carcinogenic properties. MDA has been frequently used for many years as a biomarker for lipid peroxidation of omega-3 and omega-6 fatty acids because of its facile reaction with thiobarbituric acid"[351]

Kapusta A, Kuczyńska B, Puppel K (2018) Relationship between the degree of antioxidant protection and the level of malondialdehyde in high-performance Polish Holstein-Friesian cows in peak of lactation. PLoS ONE 13 (3): e0193512. https://doi.org/10.1371/journal.pone.0193512

Acrolein

One of the most reactive molecules that can be created from fish oils is acrolein. Acrolein is more prevalently formed from fish oil than from omega-6[352][353] and does not require high temperatures to be created. Acrolein was known to be highly toxic back in 1943 when acrolein was injected in a sesame oil solvent in mice. It was shown that mice became excited, went into shock, and died within a short time frame[354]. Acrolein is used as a long-term oxidative marker for increased chances for atherosclerosis and diabetes[355]. It is implicated in the promotion of asthma[356] and inhibits testosterone production[357]. Acrolein is a small molecule and can form with many amino acids and make those proteins dysfunctional. Below is a short description of 2 molecules interacting. Acrolein can get attached to the amino acid lysine, forming N ε-(3-formyl-3,4-dehydropiperidino) lysine (FDP-lysine). FDP lysine accumulation is found in many pathologies ranging from diabetic retinopathy to stroke[358].

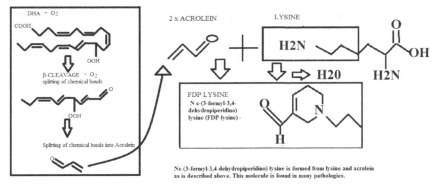

Nε-(3-formyl-3,4-dehydropiperidino) lysine is formed from lysine and acrolein as is described above. This molecule is found in many pathologies.

Nε-(3-formyl-3,4-dehydropiperidino) lysine is formed from lysine and acrolein, as is described above. This molecule is found in many pathologies.

| Isoprostanes

"This raises the question of whether n-3 derived isoprostanes/neuroprostanes and other n-3 PUFA derived oxidized fatty acids are hepatoprotective"[359]

Depner CM, Traber MG, Bobe G, Kensicki E, Bohren KM, et al. (2013) A Metabolomic Analysis of Omega-3 Fatty Acid-Mediated Attenuation of Western Diet-Induced Nonalcoholic Steatohepatitis in LDLR-/- Mice. PLoS ONE 8 (12): e83756. doi:10.1371/journal.pone.0083756

Isoprostanes are similar to prostaglandins but are made from PUFAs without the help of enzymes. Although most of the research has focused on the derivatives from omega-6, there are omega-3 isoprostanes and neuroprostanes that have been implicated in many pathologies. Because DHA usually ends up in the neurons, the DHA derivative is termed neuroprostanes. The formation into isoprostanes and neuroprostanes is a massive field as DHA alone can be converted into the F4, D4, E4, and J4 neuroprostanes. These molecules can be very dangerous and can accumulate. One of the most stable end products is F4 neuroprostanes.

"Increased cellular C20-22 n-3 PUFA promoted lipid peroxidation and thus isoprostane formation"[360]

Depner CM, Traber MG, Bobe G, Kensicki E, Bohren KM, et al. (2013) A Metabolomic Analysis of Omega-3 Fatty Acid-Mediated Attenuation of Western Diet-Induced Nonalcoholic Steatohepatitis in LDLR-/- Mice. PLoS ONE 8 (12): e83756. doi:10.1371/journal.pone.0083756

F4-Neuroprostane

"Measurement of F4-NPs, the stable product of free radical damage to DHA, also provides valuable data in exploring the role of oxidative stress in neurodegenerative diseases. The products of the IsoP pathway were found to have strong biological actions and therefore may participate as physiological mediators of the disease"[361]

Miller E, Morel A, Saso L, Saluk J. Isoprostanes and neuroprostanes as biomarkers of oxidative stress in neurodegenerative diseases. Oxid Med Cell Longev. 2014;2014:572491. doi:10.1155/2014/572491

The measurements of isoprostanes are seen by many researchers as the gold standard to assess stress levels in many pathologies, in which the isoprostane formed from AA is the most studied and well known. The DHA nonenzymatic derivatives of DHA are named neuroprostanes, as DHA is high in the brain compared to their intake. F-4 neuroprostane seems to be the most studied and most easily formed[362] (there are at least 128 isomers). These isoprostanes can cross-link with proteins, which are often found in brain diseases. F-4 neuroprostanes are found to be higher in different parts of the brain compared to healthy controls (especially the inferior parietal lobule and the sulcus middle temporal gyrus)[363]. Furthermore, neuroprostanes stop the proteasomes from removing the faulty proteins, thereby decreasing any real chance of improving the condition[364]. The amount of F4- neuroprostane is related to the severity of the disease[365].

Enzymatic Peroxidation

Beyond the breakdown of unsaturated fats when its degradation is initiated by radicals, PUFAs can also be metabolized by enzymes into eicosanoids and other products. Eicosanoids is the collective name given to the four families of chemical messengers - prostaglandins, prostacyclins, thromboxanes, and leukotrienes. All these molecules have a manifold of functions in the body. Within the literature, there is a reasonably consistent view that the omega-3 eicosanoids are anti-inflammatory, and the omega-6 is inflammatory. The picture emerges that these two omegas (3&6) fit nicely together and result in good health. These eicosanoids are formed by 3 families of enzymes (LOX, COX, and Cytochrome P450 monooxygenases). The body of literature on enzymatic peroxidation is immense, and, I would argue, mostly unknown. Below is a very short description of the different non-peroxidative products:

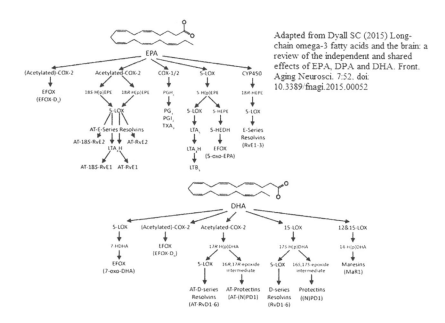

Adapted from Dyall SC (2015) Long-chain omega-3 fatty acids and the brain: a review of the independent and shared effects of EPA, DPA and DHA. Front. Aging Neurosci. 7:52. doi: 10.3389/fnagi.2015.00052

Jumping The Gun

While the case for fish oil was being made in the 1980s with claims ranging from it being the missing link between heart disease with nutrition and overall heart health, researchers began in-depth research into the enzymatic products of omega-3. The agriculture services strongly cautioned the use of omega-3 for the general public as the effects of fish oils were (and I argue still are) mostly unknown. At the time the first omega-3 supplements were being sold, the messenger products from fish oils were barely known. For example, PGE3 can be formed from EPA and thereby stops the conversion of PGE2 from AA. Since PGE2 is implicated in many pathologies, any substance that blocks this could be regarded as healthy. PGE3 is seen as less unhealthy and sometimes promoted as healthy. However, PGE3 has many of the same adverse effects as PGE2 (PGE3, for example, can increase permeability and can disrupt barrier function)[366]. While PGE3 was barely being explored, fish oils were pushed on the market and sold. It was noted that:

"PGE3 is a hormone-like substance which metabolically derives from EPA. The physiological activity of PGE3 is largely unknown. Therefore, this new finding is an implicit warning against the uncontrolled use of marine oil concentrate by the general public because some of the biological consequence of such use may not be desirable"[367]

SCIENTISTS AND THEIR SPECIALTIES Beltsville. Human Nutrition Research Center. W. Mertz, Director. Beltsville Agricultural Research Center-East Beltsville, Maryland, 20705. SPRING 1987

| LOX, COX, And Monooxygenases

As with the desaturase enzymes, the LOX, COX, and the monooxygenase system come with a host of problems and pathologies[368][369]. It gets tricky to separate the omega-3 and omega-6 pathways and effects within disease models. For example, inhibition of omega-6 eicosanoids by omega-3 can result in favorable outcomes (as with the desaturase enzymes).

When instead of focusing on only the typical omega-6 eicosanoids, but also including the omega-3 eicosanoids in eye disease research, it was found that DHA and EPA enzymatic products were increased in older people and increased with the severity of eye diseases[370]. Prostacyclin production was reduced during a low-fat diet compared to a high-fat diet regardless of supplementation with n-3 fatty acids. N-3 fatty acids stimulated the synthesis of modest amounts of thromboxane A3 and prostacyclin I3, on both the low and high saturated-fat diets[371]. Prostacyclin infusion in patients with pulmonary veno-occlusive disease can lead to death[372].

Resolving The Issues

One group of molecules that are in the spotlight right now are the resolvins. Resolvins are a family of molecules with diverse actions and are researched in light of anti-inflammatory properties. I think the pharmaceutical industry would like to manufacture these compounds directly, bypassing the omega-3 conversion. The research with these molecules is just getting started, and already difficulties are being seen.

For example, EPA can follow the P450 pathway that leads into RvE1 - while under the direction of aspirin, DHA can be turned into RvD1 by the different lipoxygenase enzymes. When mice are exposed to a brain injury, and they are treated before and after the injury with RvE1, DvD1 or saline solution, the results showed that a limited difference was seen between DvD1 and the saline solution on mortality (27% vs. 33%) but saw a 50% death rate in the RvE1 group![373]

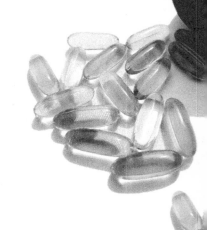

CHAPTER 6

The Making Of A Supplement

Marine oils had many purposes during the 19th century. While whale oil was the favorite, fish oil was seen as inferior. Whale oil was sold by the gallons in the early 19th century, but after the 1850s, whales became scarce, and new sea and/or new oils had to be discovered.

"In 1850 there were engaged in the whale fishery upwards of seven hundred ships, brigs, and schooners belonging to the United States, and in 1882, not one hundred are left... The oil of fish was often washed out or trown away to feed the birds serounding the fishermans boat"[374]

DeBlois, E. T. 1882. The origin of the menhaden industry. Bull. U.S. Fish Comm. 1: 46-51

Around 1921, captains found that the places where fish oil was washed away showed less rust, and the fisheries found that fish oil could be used industrially. Research conducted in the US regarding fish oil within the fisheries was first conducted in 1921 at the Washington laboratories, to identify the content of the fish oils. The work was never published, but research continued with an emphasis on menhaden oil due to the quantities that could be obtained. Until 1930, most of the research was conducted into fish liver oil. Fish liver oil had been used since the 1840s for many ailments. Until the 1920s, it was found that vitamins A and D were mostly the factors responsible for health. Research conducted in 1930 till the 1950s consistently found that fish oil "outperformed" vegetable oils in the rate and total oxidative qualities[375].

After World War II, the growth of the population and demand for food increased the need for fish products and oils. The cheapness of fish oils compared to seed-oil and lard increased its demand for livestock (mostly hydrogenated), and for industrial purposes such as varnish paints and soap overall increased its popularity. Fish oil was treated freely as an ingredient in different kinds of foodstuff. Fish oils were cheaper than other fats and were part of shortening, margarine, and other cooking oils. Outside the United States, these fish oils were mostly hydrogenated and deodorized. This process makes fish oils more saturated. Fish oils in foodstuff were quickly abandoned after the 1938 Food, Drug, and Cosmetic Act.

This act imposed stricter laws on what is considered an adulteration of foods. This act led oil manufacturers and food manufacturers to think twice before adding fish oils to food. The commercial fisheries industry was wondering what to do with the vast amounts of fish oil. The industry started out experimenting with services for paint, varnish, in the leather industry, and as an ingredient in insecticides (see picture below).

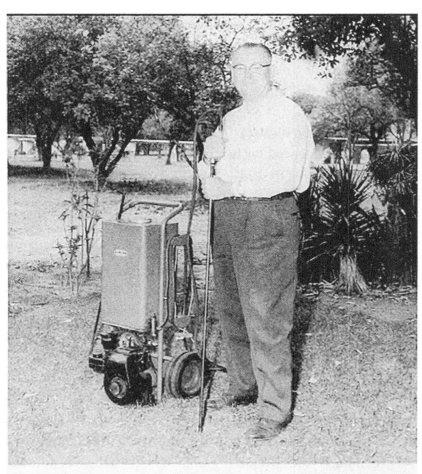

Experimental pump and probe disigned to introduce fish oil nematocides into the ground surrounding the roots of citrus trees threatened by the "spreading-decline" nematode.

From: Commercial Fisheries Review, Vol. 18, No 7. July 1956.

The synthetics, however, were outperforming the fish oils in the leather industry, while pesticides gained popularity. Around the world, countries produced more fish protein, offal, and oil. The surplus of fish oil combined with less demand from Europe left the USA commercial fishing industry worried. Vast amounts of fish oil were thrown out.

"Over 6 million pounds of potential fish oil were discarded as offal from Alaska salmon canneries this year. This loss of over a third of a million dollars in possible income from the oil alone is primarily due to the....highly perishable nature of the salmon waste, and the relatively low price brought by the crude fish oil."[376]

COMMERCIAL FISHERIES REVIEW.Vol. 17, No. 2 FEBRUARY 1955 FISH and WILDLIFE SERVICE United States Department of the Interior Washington DC

The decline of USA fish oil export in 1957 was 17% compared to the previous year, mostly because of the decrease in imports from the Netherlands and West Germany[377]. In 1957 the fisheries expected that the future of non-edible fish oil would serve as an insecticide and fungicide. The industry thought that unless new nutritional functions could be exploited, non-edible uses would be the future. Especially when, after World War II, vegetable oils started to replace fish oil in margarine, fisheries started to project possible outcomes. It was noted:

"Should unanticipated develo(p)ments upset or eliminate this market, new uses would have to be found for fish oils, or they would undergo a drastic reduction in price. The present research program of the U. S. Bureau of Commercial Fisheries is aimed at developing uses for fish

oil that could replace the European margarine market, should this become necessary."[378]

COMMERCIAL FISHERIES REVIEW. June 1958. Vol. 20, No.6 parentheses (p) are added by the author

The answer for the fisheries came from the United States 1954 public law 644 (83rd congress), which became known as the Saltonstall-Kennedy act (S-K act). The act contributed millions of dollars to achieve the goals ranging from counting methods and racial characteristics for many kinds of sea species. Furthermore, the act also made $170,000 available for new uses of fish oil[379]. The problem of fish oil was its many double bonds, which resulted in extreme vulnerability. To find a possible use for fish oil, it was figured that the negative aspects of fish oil (many double bonds) made them unique and should be further researched.

"in many cases, the characteristics of fish oils even are considered a distinct disadvantage...instead of trying to overcome the alleged disadvantages of fish oils in order to make them competitive with animals and vegetable oils, Bureau chemist decided to take advantage of these unique properties and to investigate their potential for the manufacture of industrial and pharmaceutical products"[380]

COMMERCIAL FISHERIES REVIEW, Vol. 20, No.6. June 1958.

Their unique properties, such as their unsaturation and length, were also noted to be investigated for their potential use in pharmaceutical products.

"But, in many cases, fish oils are less desirables than other organic oils, primairy because they are chemically less stable and more likely to turn rancid. For the past three years, the U.S. Bureau of commercial Fisheries and other groups have worked to develop new uses for fish oils.... Meanwhile, other laboratories continue to work on other applications for fish oils and on improved processing techniques. Possible new applications include the use of fish oils in fungicites, insecticides, pharmaceuticals for coronary disease, and heat-resistant paints"[381]

COMMERCIAL FISHERIES REVIEW. Vol. 21, No.1. January 1959

S & K STUDIES

The initial fish oil feeding experiments were found to increase: encephalomalacia (softening of the brain), also known as crazy chick disease; mortality (the addition of vitamin E avoided most of these conditions); yellow fat disease (steatites); and bad odor[382]. Fish oils were found to decrease growth[383]. This decrease in growth is probably related to the highly oxidizing nature of the fats (rancid fat can impair growth)[384]. Instead of focusing on decreasing rancidity, a lot of research went in to mask the flavor and/or odor.

Some Experiments With Fish Oil

The newly found funds were put to use. They resulted in 21 original projects: 12 projects investigating the structure and reactivity of fish oils, while 9 focussed on practical applications. One of the first experiments was conducted on swine. Fish oil was given in different quantities (5, 10, and 15% of total fats) were fed to pigs, and the 10 and 15% groups resulted in yellow fat disease, while even the 5% showed a distinct fishy smell. The polymerized fish oils, however, did not have a scent, and it was concluded that polymerized fish oil outperformed fresh fish oil from a practical perspective[385].

The Commercial Fisheries saw the massive potential for controlling vast quantities of resources. They thought this potential had to be exploited under the banner of conservation. The Fisheries saw conservatism as a means of exploitation when it came to a living resource, while nonliving resources were seen as non-renewable, and their exploitation was limited. Fish oil was a potential goldmine

"If continuing research further establishes the essentially of some of the unsaturated fatty acids peculiar to fish, the advantages of eating fish can then be more specifically stressed for nutrition in which such fatty acids are important. If fish oils are practically the only natural source of the more highly unsaturates.., our studies on the characteristics of the fatty acids will have been well founded and profitable indeed."[386]

COMMERCIAL FISHERIES REVIEW July 1958, Vol. 20 nr. 7

Finding A Market

The United States Fisheries had a significant interest in the common market to sell its products. Before the common market of Europe, the Netherlands and Germany were the most significant importers of fish oil, especially for margarine. Their sales to Europe began to decrease due to the increase in vegetable/seed oils. These fish oils were hydrogenated and, depending on the price of fish oil, were used only in minor percentages of fats used. If fish oils were used, it was for low-grade margarine. In Germany top margarine advertised with the slogan:

"CONTAINS NO FISH OIL"[387]

COMMERCIAL FISHERIES REVIEW, Volume 21, April, No. 1, 1959

To find a potential use for fish oil, it was figured that the negative aspects of fish oil (many double bonds) made them unique and should be further researched. The unique properties like their unsaturation and length were noted to be investigated for their potential use in pharmaceutical products. The fisheries thought about "aggressively" putting strategies in place for the idea that "fish oils are uniquely well fortified with more of the unsaturated fatty acids than are vegetable fats or land-animal fats"[388]. By talking about enrichment, essential, fortified, and uniqueness, terms like peroxibility, rancidity and oxidation could be largely ignored. If fish oil could be seen as special food, marketing the product could be easy. Again, the fisheries noted:

"Previous investigations have shown that fish oils have special properties which could give them a decided marketing edge. Fish oils contain a high proportion of long-chain highly-unsaturated fatty acids. The fatty acids of salmon-egg oil, particularly, are very highly unsaturated. These highly-unsaturated fatty acids may offer unique possibilities as chemical building blocks for the preparation of commercial chemical products"[389]

COMMERCIAL FISHERIES REVIEW. Vol. 17, No. 2 FEBRUARY 1955

"Since one of the unique features of fish oils is their high degree of unsaturation, it is logical that we employ that unique property to the fullest extent."[390]

COMMERCIAL FISHERIES REVIEW. April 1958. Vol. 20, No. 4.

Fish Oil As An Anti-Cholesterol Drug

Although initially it was thought that fish oils were not suitable for humans, the feeding of animals provided a potential market[391]. Two years later, studies from the S-K Act and the University of California showed the dangers of fish oil by examining the effects of fish oil on proteins and finding the browning of proteins that resembled ceroids that were found in the arteries of humans[392]. The toxicity of fish oil was further established in 1960 when the University of California found that rats fed fish oil showed growth retardation and diarrhea[393]. These and many more studies did not discourage scientists from trying to find a link between fish oils and health. As early as the mid-1950s, the link between omega-3 and heart health was made. From 1957 onwards, the S-K act financed fish oil studies regarding heart health[394]. Around this time, researchers find out that unsaturated fats lowered cholesterol. The fisheries spent no time jumping on board the cholesterol hearth health link.

"Since the study of the efficiency of these unsaturated fatty acids in lowering blood -serum cholesterol will move hand in hand with the study on the nutritional essentiality of them, our work will allow us to keep abreast of the best present thinking by medical science.

We therefore also can build on what may be found by other research workers with other fats."[395]

COMMERCIAL FISHERIES REVIEW. July 1958, Vol. 20 nr. 7

The cholesterol theory added significance to fish oils as being essential and unique. Fish oil was found to be more effective in depressing cholesterol levels than vegetable oils[396]. The fisheries noticed the importance of the cholesterol theory for the marketing of fish oils.

"But if such research is completed successfully, it may be possible to produce and market a fish-oil fatty acid for use as a means of adjusting cholesterol levels in the blood with a minimum of caloric intake"[397]

COMMERCIAL FISHERIES REVIEW. Vol. 22, No.7 July 1960.

"Research now under way will accurately pinpoint which of the unsaturated fatty acids are present in fish oils, indicate the degree of essentially of each of these acids in fat metabolism, and throw further light on the effects of inclusion of these fatty acids in the diet on the deposition of cholesterol in the arteries."[398]

COMMERCIAL FISHERIES REVIEW. July 1958. Vol 20. No. 7

A Man With A Mission

One of the researchers in the field of fish oil in the 1940s was Maurice Stansby. Before working for the Northern Oceanic and Atmospheric Agency, Stansby noted many adverse effects of fish oils[399] and even designed a test for measuring rancidity levels. After being employed for the NOAA, Stansby's primary focus changed from the negative aspects of fish to the positive aspects. The work of Stansby was deemed so important that he received the presidential award for distinguished federal civilian service (the highest honor for civilian service in the United States). Stansby, who was a director of the Seattle Technological Laboratory from 1942-1966, was mainly focused on fish oils by themselves instead of the traditional health properties of fish such as cod liver oils, proteins, etc. Under the direction of Stansby, the Seattle Laboratory started to research the cholesterol effects of fish oils but decided to outsource it to the Hormel Institute at the University of Minnesota under the direction of Walter Lundberg (who was later succeeded by James Peifer). The Hormel Institute became the expertise center. This was because fish oils were used to concentrate iron ores, and Minnesota was the iron mining capital of the USA. California University mostly conducted the food and marine sciences because of its extensive facilities. Most of the research was held along the lines of fish oils as a cholesterol depressant[400].

The Research Paid Off

After the initial sale of omega-3 in the United States, revenue increased by 600% within 3 years. The statements made by the fish oil sellers were so outlandish that in the United States,

regulatory agencies reportedly threatened to classify fish oils as drugs. This classification as a drug would mean expensive trials and research. This led to a loss of revenue to the omega-3 industry until it had a strong comeback in the 1990s and has exploded in the last 20 years.

CHAPTER 7

I n the introduction, it was noted that fish oil in the diet would often lead to a reduced intake of calories and that this, in turn, would have health-promoting effects. One of the reasons a nutritionally adequate, low-calorie diet works is the reduction of damage to cells and/or tissues. In the last century, one of the most consistent hallmarks of damage is age spots. Age spots can also be termed lipo-pigments. Lipo-pigments are the by-products of human metabolism that can accumulate in time. The term 'lipo' tells us that it is derived from lipids. These pigments are known as age spots and are toxic and fluorescent. These spots on the outside are also inside the body, especially in the areas that have a high lipid content (the nervous system and brain) and seem to accumulate in the liver. The lipopigments can be divided into at least two types: ceroids and lipofuscin.

Ceroids

Around 1883, Schultz theorized that pigmentation of human ganglion cells increased with age. In 1889, White showed that pigmentation in human ganglion cells was more frequent than in other mammals. In 1894, Goebel noticed ceroid-like products in the digestive smooth muscle of human digestive systems[401]. That same year, Hodge showed by examining the cells of the cerebrum, cerebellum, and cervical spinal cord of individuals ranging from infants to the elderly, that in young specimens, no pigment was found. At the same time, pigmentation was present in the elderly. It took about 50 years before the name ceroid was coined in 1941 by Lillie, Ashburn, Sebrell, Daft, and Lowry. These scientists described ceroid as a yellow-like lipoid pigment that occurs in the cirrhotic livers of choline-deficient rats. Before this, other scientists found that low protein favored the accumulation of ceroids[402], and that the addition of unsaturated fats observed the most significant collection of ceroids. Alpha-tocopherol (vitamin E) was found to protect and delay the onset of ceroids, even after the addition of cod liver oil. Throughout 1940-1950, studies accumulated and showed that pigmentation was associated with aging.

"It is well understood that Lipofuscin pigmentation is one of the most important characteristics of aging"[403]

Heidary F, Vaeze Mahdavi MR, Momeni F, Minaii B, Rogani M, Fallah N, et al. (2008) Food Inequality Negatively Impacts Cardiac Health in Rabbits. PLoS ONE 3 (11): e3705. https://doi.org/10.1371/journal.pone.0003705

In the 1950s and 1960s, it was found that fish oils were superior in the formation of ceroid[404][405]. The reason pigmentation occurred was theorized about after it was found that the pigmentation consisted of transition metals, proteins, and unsaturated fats. In-vitro experimentation showed that ceroid-like material could be produced with unsaturated fatty acids. Discussion occurred around the fact that the intake of unsaturated fatty acids in the diet could severely influence the rate of pigmentation forming. At the same time, saturated fats were found to be inert[406]. *The accumulation of ceroids was found in humans in the aorta, blood vessels, lymph gland, spleen, liver, adrenals, kidneys, testis, seminal vesicles, ovary, uterus, skeletal muscle, pituitary gland, and central nervous system (ganglion cells, cortex, thalamus, medulla, spinal cord, microglia, and oligodendroglia)[407]. The research went further, and it was found that fish-eating (especially fermented fish) population had an abundance of ceroids in the intestines[408]. The ceroids were found in plaques in all the different layers that are thought to form the plaque.*

| Lipofuscin

"In long-lived post-mitotic cells, autophagolysosomes (autolysosomes) progressively accumulate oxidatively modified proteins and lipids, which form a polymeric and undegradable substance called lipofuscin"[409]

Perše M, Injac R, Erman A (2013) Oxidative Status and Lipofuscin Accumulation in Urothelial Cells of Bladder in Aging Mice. PLoS ONE 8 (3): e59638. https://doi.org/10.1371/journal.pone.0059638

The brief quotation above describes how lipofuscin is formed. As the ceroids are found almost all over the body, lipofuscin is mostly found in postmitotic cells (heart, nerve, and brain cells)[410] but also in organs that have a lot of unsaturated fats, predominantly in the liver, retina, and adrenals. These cells are thought to mature and are incapable of mitosis (a division of the nucleus to produce copies). It has been shown that the iron-induced non-enzymatically oxidizing lipids (mainly unsaturated fats) attack proteins that form dysfunctional products, possibly leading to lipofuscin[411]. Research from 1984 shows that when rats were fed different fat sources (olive, lard, control, and sunflower), the lard contained more DHA than the other fat sources. Looking at the number of lipofuscins in the brain, there was no difference found between sunflower and olive oil, but the number of lipofuscins was significantly increased with the lard. It was concluded that the increase in lipofuscin was associated with 22:6 (DHA) content in the hippocampus and not with the gross peroxidation of the fat source[412]. They have shown that estrogen can increase lipofuscin formation[413].

Lysosomes are the garbage disposal sites in the cell. This organelle contains enzymes that degrade unwanted materials. Because lipofuscin cannot be (readily) degraded and can build up inside the cell, enlargement and structural disorganization of the mitochondria can result. This can result in decreased energy production seen in many pathologies[414]. Decreased mitochondria function results in the reduced capacity of lysosomal function[415]. While the lysosomal enzymes still work on trying to degrade lipofuscin, they cannot be working on other products[416]. Beyond the formation of lipofuscin, fish oils can impair lysosomes by reducing its stability, even with adequate vitamin E[417]. Lipofuscin in the hippocampus is associated with a decline in learning and memory[418]. DHEA and testosterone were found to be protective against lipid peroxidation and lipofuscin formation[419][420]. Temperature is of great importance in the accumulation of lipofuscin, as it was shown that the amount of lipofuscin was almost doubled when fish were compared at 20°C to 30°C[421]. This shows again that fish oils are not suitable for high (er) temperatures.

Yellow Fat Disease

The research continued from the 1940s into the 1950s and found that polyunsaturated fats, especially fish oils, caused yellow fat disease[422][423]. The yellow fat disease was seen as a vitamin E deficiency. Its symptoms included anorexia, muscular dystrophy, fever, flaky skin, inflamed adipose tissue, and accumulation of lipofuscin in fatty tissue.

Significant outbreaks occurred around the world in poultry and cattle that were mainly fed canned fish. It was described early on as:

- Enlarged abdomen and edema
- Loss of tone in muscles
- Black, tarry diarrhea
- Rolls of yellow fat with hemorrhages frequently around them
- Gelatinous exudate watery fluid between flesh and pelt[424]

Later studies found that under many conditions, the results of fresh or oxidized fish oils were the same in vitamin E deficient animals regarding yellow fat disease and lipofuscin[425]. The yellow fat disease is an extreme condition in which edema is common. This edema is likely the result of extreme leakiness of the cell membrane and de-energized state of the cells.

Lipofuscin Is Immunosuppressive

In the 1970s, it was suggested that the linolenic acid, EPA, and DHA (omega-3) are solely responsible for the yellow fat disease. It was concluded that yellow fat disease is associated with a steady accumulation of lipofuscin in the reticuloendothelial tissue of the liver, spleen, and lymph nodes. The reticuloendothelial system is a part of the immune system that focuses on phagocytosis, processing antigen and antibody production, the breakdown of aging red blood cells, and the storage and circulation of iron. With the accumulation of lipofuscin in the reticuloendothelial system, the immune function is reduced[426]. The reduction of the immune system is one way that fish oils promote its "positive" functions.

Longevity And The Long Chain Fatty Acids

Limiting long unsaturated chain fatty acids limits lipid peroxidation; in turn, limiting peroxidation is linked to longevity[427]. Mice whose membranes are resistant to lipid peroxidation (fewer unsaturated fats) live longer. The biggest difference in these longer-living mice is that they have less omega-3 (DHA)[428]. Looking at a database of 42 different species, it was found that as the ratio of omega-3 to omega-6 increased, lifespan decreased, and no association between DHA and longevity was found[429]. Low membrane polyunsaturation (also omega-3) slows aging[430], and fewer double bonds are associated with longevity. Besides membranes, the fatty acids in the blood show similar results. A study including humans and 10 other mammalian species analyzing the fatty acid profile found increased longevity in species with a decrease in plasma long-chain free fatty acids, double bonds, and less of the DHA-derived product 10-hydroxy-DHA[431]. As with many other organisms, a high PUFA environment (both omega-3 and -6) can cause a lot of accumulated damage.

"Altogether, the lipidome of aged worms, with a lower PC and higher polyunsaturated TG species, may reflect the

accumulation of oxidative damage in aged animals."[432]
(PC = phosphatidylcholines)

Wan, Qin-Li & Yang, Zhong-Lin & Zhou, Xiao-Gang & Ding, Ai-Jun & Pu, Yuanzhu & Luo, Huai-Rong & Wu, Gui-Sheng. (2019). The Effects of Age and Reproduction on the Lipidome of Caenorhabditis elegans. Oxidative Medicine and Cellular Longevity. 2019. 1-14. 10.1155/2019/5768953.

In centenarians (people living longer than 100 years), a study from Italy was set up to see the differences between the young, elderly, and the centenarians. The observations showed a decreased level of EPA and fully functioning anti-oxidative systems in the centenarians versus the elderly[433].

The number of double bonds seems more important than the total of polyunsaturated fats. The increase in polyunsaturated fats can decrease the total amount of double bonds. The parent linoleic acid has two double bonds and does not increase the ratio as much as DHA which has six double bonds[434]. From this standpoint, 3 grams of linoleic acid equals 1 gram of DHA. When krill oil and pharmaceutical fish oils were substituted for soy oil, it showed a decrease in lifespan, and an increase in tumor formation and hemorrhagic diathesis compared to controls[435]. Mice fed different kinds of fat on a low-calorie diet lived longer on a monounsaturated and saturated intake than on a fish oil diet[436]. Long-term mice studies show that males are particularly affected when taking fish oil. One study showed that while low dose omega-3 decreased longevity by 9%, high omega-3 intakes decreased lifespan by 18%[437].

"Interestingly, increased concentrations of plasma polyunsaturated fatty acids have been implicated in the pathogenesis of chronic diseases"[438]

Collino S, Montoliu I, Martin F-PJ, Scherer M, Mari D, Salvioli S, et al. (2013) Metabolic Signatures of Extreme Longevity in Northern Italian Centenarians Reveal a Complex Remodeling of Lipids, Amino Acids, and Gut Microbiota Metabolism. PLoS ONE 8 (3): e56564. https://doi.org/10.1371/journal.pone.0056564

A Bees Tale

Queen bees can live until three years, while worker bees have a maximum lifespan of a few months. The difference in lifespan became significant when it was shown that the complete set of genes (genome) of the worker bees and queen bee are the same. The difference comes primarily from nutrition[439]. When looking at the difference, it was suspected that the royal jelly was the magic food that makes the difference. However, it turns out that the royal jelly is not magical - the worker bees' diet is just many times worse. The worker bees' diet consists mostly of bee bread - a combination of jelly, honey, and stored pollen that has been fermented. Pollen contains flavonoids that are anti-fertility, and that decreases the development of ovaries[440]. Until about the 3rd day of life, both types of bees are fed royal honey, after which the worker bees are weaned off most of the royal jelly, and an increase in pollen and nectar is supplied. Most of the attention on the differences between a queen bee and a worker diet focuses on the addition of 10-hydroxy-trans-2-decenoic acid (a monounsaturated fatty acid that is high in royal jelly), but there is more to the story. The most significant differences seem to be the decrease of sugars in the workers' diet compared to their food and the increase in polyunsaturated fatty acids (also omega-3) in their diet. When sugars were added to the female worker bee at an early age, queen bees could be produced[441]. The polyunsaturated fats seem to replace mono-unsaturated fats in workers within the first week after the dietary changes. These polyunsaturated fats are incorporated into membranes and are ready to be peroxidized. It has been shown that, in line with other animals, the low membrane peroxidation of queen bees compared to worker bees can account for the difference in lifespan[442].

Naked Mole-Rat

It has been observed that the naked mole-rat lives about nine times as long as the typical mouse. When comparing the phospholipid of the two different species, remarkable differences can be seen. This is even though total phospholipids are the same, and DHA is seen in phosphatidylcholines, phosphatidylethanolamines, and phosphatidylserines (PE more than PC). The quantities, however, show a different story. As the naked mole-rat lives nine times as long as mice, the amount of DHA in mice is at least nine-fold compared to the naked mole-rat (the average is about 11 fold). Furthermore, naked mole rats have higher levels of plasmalogen in their tissues, suggesting a vital role for the peroxisomes for their longevity[443]. In bacteria, it is known that an increase in unsaturated fats decrease plasmalogen levels, as the unsaturated fats cause a disorganized cell membrane[444].

Bivalve Mollusks

Bivalve mollusks are seen as important for studying longevity. Bivalve mollusks include clams, oysters, mussels, and scallops. These sea-animals are seen as the longest living animals and can reach an age of over 500 years. The longest living species of mollusks are the Arctica islandica, which has been reported to live until 507 years of age. Compared to 4 other classes of mud clams with a maximum of 106 years, the mitochondria from Arctica islandica has less omega-3 and a considerably lower peroxidation index, making it more resistant to oxidation. One of the most obvious observations is that as DHA decreases in the mitochondria, lifespan increases[445].

Double Bonds Equals Double Trouble

"The rate of mitochondrial ROS production, extent of mtDNA (but not nuclear DNA) oxidative damage, and degree of membrane fatty acid unsaturation (a determinant of vulnerability to lipid peroxidation) are all inversely correlated with longevity across species"[446]

Kujoth GC, Bradshaw PC, Haroon S, Prolla TA (2007) The Role of Mitochondrial DNA Mutations in Mammalian Aging. PLoS Genet 3 (2): e24. https://doi. org/10.1371/journal.pgen.0030024

Beyond the peroxide index, the factors associated with the unsaturation of fats also seem crucial for not reaching longevity potential. The before mentioned desaturase enzymes are minimized in animals that live long, resulting in a low unsaturation index[447][448]. With the desaturase enzymes, there usually follows beta-oxidation to shorten the unsaturated fatty acid to DHA. Beta-oxidation is very limited in animals with extreme longevity[449]. Estrogen can upregulate desaturase enzymes (chapter 3). Comparing testosterone, DHT and estrogen between 2 (older) age groups, there was a massive drop in free-testosterone (20%) and free-DHT (20%) and an enormous increase in free estrogen (30%) in the oldest group compared to the younger group[450].

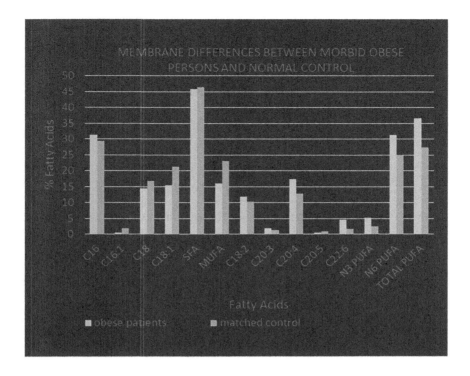

Data were taken from Genio, Gianmattia. (2015). Morbid Obesity is Associated to Altered Fatty Acid Profile of Erythrocyte Membranes. Journal of Diabetes & Metabolism. 06. 10.4172/2155-6156. 1000582.

This chart shows the differences in membranes fatty acid content from morbidly obese versus the control group. Note the significant differences between mono-unsaturated fats. The data goes on to explain that omega-3 fatty acid is doubled in obese patients compared to the control group. At the same time, omega-6 is moderately increased in obese patients. It seems that longevity is associated with more saturated cell-membranes. In comparing membranes from offspring from the general population with offspring from centenarians, the difference was noticeable in the peroxidation index. The progeny of centenarians had higher amounts of monounsaturated fat and decreased amounts of polyunsaturated fats[451]. When red blood cells from centenarians are compared to the control, it was shown that they have an increase in the actin protein structure as part of the cytoskeleton and a sturdy organizational structure. Omega-3 has been shown to decrease the genes for actin production, leading to a reduction in actin volume, which is a loss in muscle volume[452].

Fish Oil Lowers Vitamin E

Vitamin E has many functions in the human body, often working in the opposite direction to fish oil[453]. For example, Interferon-γ and interleukin -2 are part of the immune system and are subsequently increased by vitamin E and decreased by fish oils[454][455]. The total amount of double bonds in the membrane is called the peroxidation index. Fish oils were compared with alpha-linolenic and linoleic acid with regards to lipid peroxidation in vitro and in vivo in monkey livers. The results showed that fish oils outperformed the other lipids in lipid peroxidation, lipofuscin, and glutathione-peroxidase activity. Besides, vitamin E did not do well against fish oil compared to the other oils[456]. When cod liver oil is compared with lard in rats on a vitamin E deficiency, it becomes clear that cod liver oil and fish oil are more efficient in the destruction of vitamin E than lard[457]. Of different oils tested, fish oil proved to affect vitamin E levels the most[458].

In 1920, while investigating if milk was the perfect food, Henry Albright Mattill found that rats' growth declined, and females were unable to produce offspring. After experimentation with wheat germ oil, his team found that vitamin X (vitamin E) reduced the uptake of oxygen when compared to the subjects without vitamin X and prevented rancidity[459]. The different vitamers of vitamin E were named tocopherols after the Greek (toco = birth; ferein

= bringing). After many studies, it was found that rats needed vitamin E to produce offspring successfully. Vitamin E is seen as the primary antioxidant mechanism in fat tissue systems. Vitamine E can stop and absorb the lipid-free radicals leading to a break in the propagation phase. It is therefore known as a chain breaker. It is thought that the lipid generated free radical is more attracted to vitamin E than the unsaturated fatty acids, stopping the chain reaction. As peroxidation of unsaturated fish oils uses up vitamin E, any excess of unsaturated fats or not enough vitamin E can leave peroxidation unchecked (depending on the other chain-breakers). It was found that exclusion of vitamin E caused encephalomalacia (softening of the brain) in poultry, leading to 'crazy chick disease,' and could destroy vitamin A, B complex, Vitamin C, and Vitamin E[460].This is important because it was later found that, for example, vitamin A can protect the brain mitochondria against induced lipid peroxidation (more potent than some of the vitamin E isomers)[461]. In the 1940s, a vitamin E deficiency was seen by a scientist as the same as a cod liver oil or rancid fat diet[462].

Cell Fluidity

"The structure and organization of the cell membrane are central to many biological functions, and although they have been extensively studied, there is still much that we don't understand."[463]

Nickels JD, Chatterjee S, Stanley CB, Qian S, Cheng X, Myles DAA, et al. (2017) The in vivo structure of biological membranes and evidence for lipid domains. PLoS Biol 15 (5): e2002214. https://doi.org/10.1371/journal.pbio.2002214

"Although different cell membrane models have been introduced over the past century, we are still far from fully understanding this important cellular component"[464]

Zhao W, Tian Y, Cai M, Wang F, Wu J, Gao J, et al. (2014) Studying the Nucleated Mammalian Cell Membrane by Single Molecule Approaches. PLoS ONE 9 (5): e91595. https://doi.org/10.1371/journal.pone.0091595

One often-cited reason for supplementing omega-3 is that these fatty acids are incorporated into the membrane of the cell and that they increase its fluidity[465]. Membrane fluidity is thought to be conducive to cell function. With the necessary fluidity, it is believed that proper transport, receptors, and metabolism are assured. Membrane function, importance, and even existence are heavily debated and extremely complex. It is estimated that at any time, there are 1500 different lipid arrangements and more than 100 different proteins that can change at every microsecond. While this sounds very complex and random, recent investigations find that the membrane is more nonrandom and symmetrical than previously assumed, with a more important role for the proteins and less for the lipids.

"New evidence, however, shows that the distribution of proteins is not random and that lateral diffusion is restricted by the interaction of the membrane-bound receptors with cytoskeleton or cytosolic molecules, indicating a lateral heterogeneity in the membranes"[466]

Zhao W, Tian Y, Cai M, Wang F, Wu J, Gao J, et al. (2014) Studying the Nucleated Mammalian Cell Membrane by Single Molecule Approaches. PLoS ONE 9 (5): e91595. https://doi.org/10.1371/journal.pone.0091595

"Thus, cell membrane structure should be considered "mosaic", i.e., an assemblage of small pieces, and not "fluid", as emphasized in the dynamically structured mosaic model"[467]

Zhao W, Tian Y, Cai M, Wang F, Wu J, Gao J, et al. (2014) Studying the Nucleated Mammalian Cell Membrane by Single Molecule Approaches. PLoS ONE 9 (5): e91595. https://doi.org/10.1371/journal.pone.0091595

This means that the fluidity of a cell membrane is less critical than previously thought. Below is a simple drawing of a cell membrane. Newer studies show that the structured view of the cell and the membrane leave a less important role for unsaturated fats.

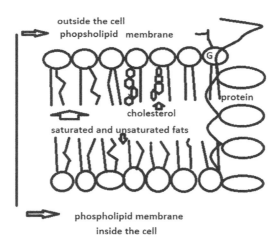

Compared to oleic acid (1 double bond), DHA has considerably different effects on the cell membrane. DHA covers a greater area in the membrane and causes increased permeability and more leakages. In the membrane, cholesterol and the unsaturated fatty acids seem to repel each other, leading to concentrated regions of either cholesterol or unsaturated fats. Research from the 1980s showed that the fluidity in the membrane from double bonds has more to do with the location of the double bond than the number of double bonds in fatty acids[468]. As the double bond is located in the middle of the fatty acid chain, it increases fluidity more than when it is located away from the center. Apart from the first double bonds, the second to sixth double bonds add little to increase fluidity; it does, however, raise the possibility to peroxidize[469], regardless of the position of the double bond (bis). As the body can synthesize up to 3 double bonds located at the center, as is the case with oleic acid, fluidity does not seem a sufficient reason to take fish oils. Furthermore, the body has mechanisms in place to keep the fluidity constant even when there is limited PUFA in the diet.

"Feeding diets rich in saturated fatty acids decreases the ratio of ω 6/ ω 3 PUFA in PL of mitochondria from rat liver, heart, or kidney, but leaves the ratio of saturated/ unsaturated fatty acyls unchanged"[470]

Hoch FL. Lipids and thyroid hormones. Prog Lipid Res. 1988;27(3):199–270. doi:10.1016/0163-7827(88)90013-6. Permission from Elsevier

The idea that increased fluidity is a good thing without discernment lacks logic. For example, these toxins can increase membrane fluidity.

- Polycyclic aromatic hydrocarbons (PAHs)[471] (protected by cholesterol feeding)
- DDT[472] (insecticide) works partly by disrupting the cell ordering properties of cholesterol.
- Polychlorinated biphenyl (PCB)[473]
- Fenvalerate (insecticide)[474]

Furthermore, an increase in fluidity in the cell membrane is associated with poorer prognosis in patients with cancer[475]. The excess fluidity can lead to a loss in cell viability[476], Prolactin[477], nitric oxide[478], and estrogen[479] can increase membrane fluidity.

Conditions that lead to an increase in fluidity can increase the likeliness of infections[480]. Infections decrease cholesterol in the cell and can make the membrane more fluid, leading to an "infectious burden"[481]. Leukocytes in the blood of Alzheimer's patients show increased fluidity compared to controls[482]. Fish oil increases the permeability of the intestinal barrier, the increased permeability of tight junction, possibly leading to cancer metastasis[483484]. One way fish oil can make the intestines more permeable is by reducing Mucin2[485]. Mucin2 is a gel-like substance offering protection for the epithelial cells.

"Patients on a long term gluten-free diet had similar intakes of EPA plus DHA compared to controls. Contrary to expectations, DHA serum levels were significantly higher in CD patients compared to healthy controls and were unrelated to MDD status."[486] CD = Celiac Disease

van Hees NJM, Giltay EJ, Geleijnse JM, Janssen N, van der Does W (2014) DHA Serum Levels Were Significantly Higher in Celiac Disease Patients Compared to Healthy Controls and Were Unrelated to Depression. PLoS ONE 9 (5): e97778. https://doi.org/10.1371/journal.pone.0097778

Fish oil can also make membranes less fluid by lipid peroxidation, as the breakdown products of fish oil can slow down functioning and make the membrane rigid[487]. The lipid peroxidation of fats makes the cell membrane more rigid than cholesterol does[488].

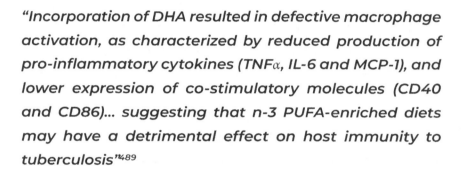

CHAPTER 8

| Anti Inflammatory Or Anti-Immune?

"Incorporation of DHA resulted in defective macrophage activation, as characterized by reduced production of pro-inflammatory cytokines (TNFα, IL-6 and MCP-1), and lower expression of co-stimulatory molecules (CD40 and CD86)... suggesting that n-3 PUFA-enriched diets may have a detrimental effect on host immunity to tuberculosis"[489]

Bonilla DL, Ly LH, Fan Y-Y, Chapkin RS, McMurray DN (2010) Incorporation of a Dietary Omega 3 Fatty Acid Impairs Murine Macrophage Responses to Mycobacterium tuberculosis. PLoS ONE 5 (5): e10878. https://doi.org/10.1371/journal.pone.0010878

"Most studies have focused on the effects of PUFAs, particularly omega-3, derived from fish oil. These omega-3 fatty acids generally inhibit immune and inflammatory functions by decreasing lymphocyte proliferation, cytokine production, NK cytotoxicity, and antibody production, among other effects...The fatty acids that most affect the immune system are those

of the omega-3 type, which has an inhibitory action, as mentioned before, followed by the omega-6 type, which mostly has a less pronounced effect."[490]

Pompéia C., Lopes L.R., Miyasaka C.K., Procópio J., Sannomiya P., Curi R.. Effect of fatty acids on leukocyte function. Braz J Med Biol Res [Internet]. 2000 Nov [cited 2020 Feb 25]; 33 (11): 1255-1268. Available from: http://www.scielo.br/scielo.php?script=sci_arttext&pid=S0100-879X2000001100001&lng=en. https://doi.org/10.1590/S0100-879X2000001100001.

In 1992, Tufts University was part of a national program to recommend a diet that would lower cholesterol to reduce heart disease. Many steps were taken to find out the primary responses when participants were fed the different foods. When added omega-3 diets, given to human volunteers were compared with controls and high omega-6 menus, the logical reduction in the PGE2 was seen as expected and reasoned to be one of the contributing factors. The team also found reduced immune responses following a high fish and low-fat diet compared to both control and high omega-6 and ALA diet. The authors reasoned that although lowered parameters of inflammation can be seen, the organism might be compromised against infections[491]. Even with a very low dose of 150 mg DHA and 30 mg, EPA immune-suppressive actions can be observed.

The idea of fish oil being anti-inflammatory comes from the comparison with omega-6. With fish oil, the inflammatory response is, in many cases, not dealt with but is somewhat lacking in any response, letting it seem to be anti-inflammatory. As described before, the actions of prostaglandins from fish oils can be partly defined as stuporous and sedentary. In this state, there seems to be reduced response to infections and accidents (longer bleeding time). In the 1980s, this immune-suppressive mechanism of fish oils started to become popular in transplantations and autoimmune diseases[492493]. There are many ways in which fish oil can lower immunity. Some of these are elucidated, while others are unknown. One way in which DHA inhibits lymphoid cells is by causing disorganization of the cell membrane, resulting in the exclusion of proteins in the membrane (probably by activating phospholipase D), resulting in impairment of the cell (DHA tends to replace palmitate, a saturated fat)[494].

Immune System

There are two main types of immune groups within the body. One group is classified as the innate immune system, and the other is the adaptive immune system. The innate immune system is rapid in responding, while the adaptive group can take days to develop a response. A function of the immune system is to protect us from more than 1000 different kinds of bacteria, worms, parasites, fungi, and viruses. A very simplistic view of the immune system is seen below.

Innate immune system	Adaptive immune system
Macrophages	CD8T Cells
Dendritic cells	Cd4T cells
Natural killer cells	B Cells
NK-T cells	Regulatory Cells
Neutrophils	NK-T Cells
Basophils	
Eosinophils	

One of the first lines of defense of the immune system and important cell defense against invaders is the macrophages. Beyond their function as sensors of the pathogen and as a communication cell for backup, they have many other vital features such as repairing and removing damaged tissue.

Macrophages

As one of the first lines of defense, the macrophages are a good indicator of immune status and longevity probability. Studies with mice show that the difference between old and long-lived mice is the lack of accumulation of lipofuscin in the macrophages of the long-lived mice compared to old mice[495]. Macrophages studies show that they have a great ability to conform to a situation and adapt. When fish oil is implemented and is incorporated into macrophages, the ability of fish oil containing macrophages to kill a tumor target is greatly diminished compared to corn oil. Furthermore, an increase in intercellular calcium mobilization is seen[496][497] - increased intercellular mobilization is associated with cell death. The diminished response and activity can be considered as an anti-inflammatory when one concentrates on one aspect instead of the bigger picture.

When one takes a step back, it can be seen that fish oils also lower the following cytokines/molecules:

PMN Polymorphonuclear cell	MACROPHAGES	T CELL	APC antigen-presenting cell	B CELL
PSGL-1	IL-1	Proliferation	MHCII	1gG2a
CD-62L	TNF ALPHA	CD62L		1Ggi
IL-8	IL-6	ICAM-1		
	IL-8	LFA-1		
TBAX 2	IL-12	CD2		
PGE2	ICAM-1	CD4		
LTB4	HMCII	Th1		
	TBAX 2	y-IFN		
	PGE2	DTH		
	LTB4	IL-2		
		Th2		
		IL-4		
		IL-6		
		IL-10		

All these molecules can be down regulated by intake of fish oils. Data taken from: Harbige, Laurence. (2003). Fatty acids, the immune response, and autoimmunity: A question of n-6 essentiality and the balance between n-6 and n-3. Lipids. 38. 323-41. 10.1007/s11745-003-1067-z.

Some more in-depth examples of immune cells that are lowered by fish oil

Interleukin 10: lowering IL-10 can result in increased mortality from infection[498]. IL-10 is anti-inflammatory and is an essential regulatory negative feedback mechanism after an immune response has been mounted[499].

Interleukin 4 and 13: IL-4 and IL-13 have many similar functions, which are diverse and, in many cases, yet to be discovered. Its functions seem to be mainly in T cell supporting functions and brain functions. When animals are absent in interleukin 4 or IL-13, learning and memory functions are adversely affected[500][501]. Infants who receive less IL-13 via breast milk have a higher incidence of atopic dermatitis[502]. When pregnant women are given fish oil, the offspring show decreased IL-4[503].

Interferons: interferons get activated by a possible pathogen and trigger the response of hundreds of host proteins. One of the key responses to block viruses, for example, is the up-regulation of cholesterol to prevent the virus from entering the cell. As fish oil lowers blood cholesterol levels, it also reduces the presence of cholesterol protein in the membrane. These proteins and cholesterol are mostly present in lipid rafts (which can contain some omega-3). When omega-3 are added to cell membranes, these lipid rafts are decreased, leading to diminished interferon response[504]. It is estimated that omega-3 can disrupt 40% of lipid rafts' clustering and size[505]. Longevity is associated with higher levels of interferons and is more responsive to stimuli to activate interferons[506]. The decrease in lipid rafts can also have other consequences as lipid rafts can contain GABA receptors; when cholesterol is decreased, GABA can become less responsive. Only the addition of cholesterol seems to restore GABA[507].

Immunoglobin A (IgA): IgA can be the first antibodies generated against an infection. Lowered IgA has been associated with increased mortality in many conditions, especially the elderly[508]. Many studies with fish oil show promise (although I do not advocate them) with conditions requiring lower immunity. Examples are organ transplants and immunoglobin A nephropathy (IgAN is a condition where immunoglobin A can get "stuck" in the kidneys and cause inflammation)[509].

Delayed-type hypersensitivity (DTH): DTH is an immune response that can take days to develop. DTH is a cell-mediated response, and fish oil supplementation shows a decrease in delayed-type hypersensitivity[510]. The reduction in DTH is often seen in immune-compromised individuals[511], and a decrease in DTH increases mortality during intensive care and trauma[512].

Besides, fish oil can up-regulate

Interleukin-5: fish oils promote IL-5[513]. It can increase the fibrosis of the liver[514].

Transforming growth factor-beta 1 (TGF-beta 1): TGF-beta 1 is increased by fish oil[515]. This is a protein that is activated and is seen as one of the main contributors to fibrosis[516], thyroid hormone opposites, and a decrease of TGF[517]. TGF-Beta is increased in cord blood of pregnant women taking fish oil[518].

Tumor necrosis factor (TNF): TNF is a protein that, as the name suggests, causes necrosis[519]. Fish oil enhances the transcription of messenger RNA (which can cause the production of TNF protein)[520].

The breakdown products of the omega-3 produce immunosuppressive actions[521522]. This can increase morbidity and mortality by lowering resistance against infections[523524525526527] and provide a variety of inflammatory mediators by macrophages[528] (this reaction is more severe than the body's own immunological memory responses[529]). This is seen even in tiny doses[530]. The immunosuppressive properties of omega-3 are thought to be useful for transplanting organs, as the lowering of the immune system decreases the chance of rejection. However, this does not always mean a better survival rate[531].

DHA increases the release of ATP in the extracellular tissue[532]. Whatever its primary function is, the release of ATP from the cell is associated with the pro-inflammatory activity. The removal of ATP from extracellular tissue can prevent cellular disintegration, mitochondrial damage, apoptosis, intestinal barrier disruption, and even mortality[533]. Extracellular ATP releases estrogen[534], and prolactin[535], thereby increasing calcium inside the cell[536]. Extracellular ATP is high in tumors but nonexistent in healthy tissue[537].

Interleukin-6

Many articles and some studies show that macrophages with fish oil, reduce interleukin 6 (IL-6). This focus solely on IL-6, and this shift in reduced IL-6 seems beneficial, as IL-6 is involved in many pathologies[538] (olive oil and coconut oil also can reduce IL-6[539540]). A diet with an absence of omega-3 and omega-6 reduces IL-6 more than omega-3 & -6[541]. Furthermore, when olive oil and fish oil (and control) are compared to pregnant animals and their offspring, the fish oil piglets and sows showed higher levels of breakdown products and higher levels of IL-6, TNF-α, as well as the increased death rate for progeny and lower milk production[542]. Many studies show that fish oil can increase rather than decrease IL-6[543544], or that no difference is shown[545].

Even though olive oil seems to be better in reducing IL-6 and TNF-alpha and healthier overall (fewer breakdown products), it has only 149 studies compared to 751 on fish oil regarding IL-6. When checking PubMed with the different interleukins IL-6, fish oil has more reviews than any other interleukin. This focus of fish oil on reducing IL-6 takes the attention away from the fact that it is increasing and decreasing another interleukin that can lower health.

SEARCH	NUMBER OF ARTICLES
Interleukin 1 and fish oil	385
Interleukin 2 and fish oil	150
Interleukin 3 and fish oil	1
Interleukin 4 and fish oil	109
Interleukin 5 and fish oil	27
Interleukin 6 and fish oil	751
Interleukin 7 and fish oil	5
Interleukin 8 and fish oil	145
Interleukin 9 and fish oil	3
Interleukin 10 and fish oil	275
Interleukin 11 and fish oil	1
Interleukin 12 and fish oil	45

Omega-3 increases in aged neutrophils, probably lessening their function. Neutrophils produce hypochlorous acid (HOCL) as part of their immune activity. HOCL is very reactive, and when it comes in contact with the unsaturated fats, it provides a host of products. When HOCL gets metabolized by the enzyme myeloperoxidase, it seems to favor the formation of chlorohydrin. Chlorohydrin is found in atherosclerotic plaques and has been suggested as a possible initiator[546]. When the same enzyme myeloperoxidase producing reactive chlorinating species attacks plasmalogen and unsaturated fatty acids, its products can link with amino acids and get attached to the arteries. It has been shown that the unsaturated lysophosphatidylcholine containing DHA was exclusively found in atherosclerotic arteries, not in healthy arteries[547].

The Other Side(s) Of The Immune System

The immune system also functions in other under-recognized, but essential areas such as clearing up of debris, non-functioning tissues, damaged cells, and wound repair. When taking this function of the immune system into account, molecules like cholesterol and platelets could have a significant and positive role instead of negative. At the same time, it leaves the omega-3 in a less favorable light.

| Platelets As Part Of The Immune System

"As a first line of host defense, platelets act as primitive immune cells, interacting with invading bacterial pathogens or recruiting immune cells"[548]

Yue L, Pang Z, Li H, Yang T, Guo L, Liu L, et al. (2018) CXCL4 contributes to host defense against acute Pseudomonas aeruginosa lung infection. PLoS ONE 13(10): e0205521. https://doi.org/10.1371/journal.pone.0205521

Fish oils have a known effect on platelet function. Platelets are small blood cells that stop bleeding and aid in repair. Omega-3 can inhibit this activation and clump together of these tiny cells. In this way, it thins the blood and can stop excessive blood clotting, but it increases bleeding. Platelets have, from a historical perspective, essential roles that focused on protecting endothelium function. Its blood clotting function was seen as "doubtful"[549]. Today, platelets are defined by their blood clotting function, not as part of the immune system. I think as fish oil suppresses the immune system, suppression of platelet function could be beneficial in certain conditions but does not seem very healthy. Platelets can interact and activate many other immune cells and link up with them to stop bacteria spreading, and can even absorb them.

Because fish oil is incorporated into platelets instead of arachidonic acid, the eicosapentaenoic acid in the membrane can be changed into thromboxane A3 and prostacyclin A3 instead of arachidonic acid that can be transformed into thromboxane A2. Thromboxane A3, compared to thromboxane A2, is a weak platelet aggregation and a vasoconstrictor.

In platelet aggregation, increased fibrinogen binding proteins increase the platelet aggravation, possibly leading to increased protection against bacteria. When aggravating promoting fibrinogen is inhibited, Staphylococcus aureus can be more lethal[550]. The effects of fish oils on platelet function can increase bleeding time. Warnings have been made against the use of fish oils over concerns about increased bleeding time[551]. In healthy people, it was recently found that fish oils have no beneficial effect on platelet function[552].

Cholesterol As Part Of The Immune System

"infected macrophages could be corrected by liposomal delivery of cholesterol indicating a possible therapeutic role of liposomal cholesterol in infection."[553]

Roy K, Mandloi S, Chakrabarti S, Roy S (2016) Cholesterol Corrects Altered Conformation of MHC-II Protein in Leishmania donovani Infected Macrophages: Implication in Therapy. PLoS Negl Trop Dis 10(5): e0004710. https://doi.org/10.1371/journal.pntd.0004710

An under-reported side of cholesterol is its anti-inflammatory function and association with the immune system. Substances that stimulate the immune system also encourage the lipoprotein system that binds to bacteria, viruses, and toxins[554][555][556][557]. Since cholesterol acts as an antioxidant[558][559][560], it seems plausible that cholesterol aids as an antioxidant to reduce inflammation. For example, right after myocardial infarction, cholesterol is decreased. After this initial decrease, the body goes into overdrive synthesizing cholesterol. This cholesterol goes into the cell, probably to aid in repair[561]. This combination of inflammatory inducers, LDL, and neutrophils aggregates and can ultimately form a plaque. Without cholesterol, these attacks on the body may be left unchecked and potentially cause more damage. Statins are used to treat CVD and seem to have benefits for the heart[562]. Still, studies also show that statins work independently from lowering cholesterol and contain anti-inflammatory properties[563][564].

Lowering LDL aggressively by statins showed the same improvements as when LDL levels remained almost unchanged[565]. Statins can work on inhibiting the overproductions of cytokines and nitric oxide[566]. The statins, like all medications, have many less favorable effects and are anti-metabolic by inhibiting or lowering mitochondria abilities[567]. Furthermore, statins can act like fish oil in suppressing the immune system[568].

"It is important to note, that not all statin-mediated changes in the cell are inherently tied to cholesterol levels. As statins inhibitory target is further upstream from cholesterol synthesis, cholesterol-independent effects may be at work as well."[569]

Bietz A, Zhu H, Xue M and Xu C (2017) Cholesterol Metabolism in T Cells. Front. Immunol. 8:1664. doi: 10.3389/fimmu.2017.01664

Fish Intake and Heart Disease

I will now explore the pre-research that led to the association of fish oil with heart health. In 1951 Strom and Jensen found that in Norway during World War II, heart attacks declined. The researchers associated the lack of saturated fat and the consumption of fish with this decline[570]. In 1953, Schornagel found the same conditions in Holland during the war.

These studies led an American scientist, Dr. Nelson, to experiment with his patients. His research spanned 20 years and found that patients who were consuming fatty fish three times a week had only a 25% chance of dying of heart disease compared to the control. At around the same time, a landmark study from Scandinavia showed that Eskimos from Greenland had a low incidence of ischaemic heart disease compared to the Danish control. The researchers proposed that the significant quantities of marine food might be contributing to this since Eskimos had lower blood lipid levels (especially pre-beta- lipoproteins)[571]. The same researchers published in 1978 that high levels of EPA might be a protective factor against thrombosis[572]. The same study found very low levels of arachidonic acid levels, but the researchers probably found this not newsworthy. As a cold fish eating country, the Dutch progressed with the epidemiologic research which accumulated in the famous 1985 Wageningen study. In 1985, Kromhout showed that 30 grams of fish per day were associated with a 50% reduction in mortality from coronary heart disease[573]. After some disappointing follow-up studies, the lead author of the original 1985 study, Kromhout, advises eating the whole fish. Kromhout suggests that the qualities of fish like vitamin D, selenium, instead of fish oil, contribute to a total package[574].

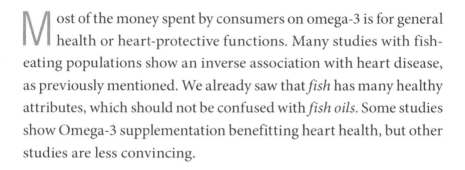

CHAPTER 9

The "Heart Healthy" Supplement

M ost of the money spent by consumers on omega-3 is for general health or heart-protective functions. Many studies with fish-eating populations show an inverse association with heart disease, as previously mentioned. We already saw that *fish* has many healthy attributes, which should not be confused with *fish oils*. Some studies show Omega-3 supplementation benefitting heart health, but other studies are less convincing.

Some examples:

- In Italy, a randomized, placebo-controlled clinical trial enrolled 860 general practitioners, 12,513 patients, men and women with multiple cardiovascular risk factors, or atherosclerotic vascular disease (excluding myocardial infarction) who were followed for five years. The patients either received 1 gram of n-3 fatty acid or a placebo (olive oil). The study found no benefit from fish oils[575].
- In the United Kingdom, a study divided 3114 men into four groups (group 1 advised to eat fatty fish or take an omega-3 capsule; group 2 encouraged to eat more vegetables, fruits,

and oats; group 3 given both types of advice; and group 4 given specific information). All men were under the age of 70 with angina showed that the group that was told to eat fatty fish or consume omega-3 capsules was worst off (especially fish oil capsule consumers) with regards to cardiac death[576].

- In the Netherlands, 4837 patients with a myocardial infarction history were placed in a double-blind, placebo-controlled trial. These patients were divided into four groups. Group 1 received margarine supplemented with 400 mg EPA/DHA; group 2 received margarine supplemented with 2 grams of ALA; group 3 received margarine supplemented with EPA/DHA and ALA, and group 4 received a margarine placebo. The study group found no effect of low dose EPA-DHA[577].

- The same group used data from the study described above following 639 patients for 40 months and again four groups were followed: group 1, control; group 2, ALA (2 grams); group 3, EPA-DHA (400 mg); group 4, EPA DHA and ALA (400mg plus 2 grams). The patients were measured on N-Terminal-pro Brain Natriuretic Peptide (NT-proBNP), a biomarker of heart failure. The results showed that the fish oil groups had "slightly" elevated levels compared to the placebo group[578]. They also found no difference comparing high-sensitivity C-reactive protein[579].

- In France, 2501 patients with a history of myocardial infarction, unstable angina, or ischaemic stroke were placed in a double-blind, randomized, placebo-controlled trial. This study also found that supplementing omega-3 had no significant effect on the reduction of major vascular events, compared to the placebo[580].

- Following 667 people for ten years in Holland, it was found that after adjustment of cofactors, they found no beneficial effects of linolenic oil regarding coronary artery disease (CAD)[581].
- In Spain, 41,091 participants who were recruited between 1992 and 1996 were again followed up on in 2004 through surveys. They found no association between EPA, DHA, and CHD[582].
- 44,895 male professionals were followed for six years through a dietary questionnaire. The food intake was translated into omega-3 content. Comparing the low omega-3 group (0.07 gram per day average) to the high omega-3 group (0.58 gram per day average), the high omega-3 group had increased CHD, myocardial cases, and more sudden deaths and nonsignificant higher mortality from CHD[583].
- After receiving 1 gram of omega-3 ethyl esters for one year versus a control group that both followed guideline adjusted treatment, it was found that survivors of acute myocardial infarction (3851 patients) showed no improvements; in fact, the omega-3 group showed a non-significant increase in mortality, neoplasms, and the need for therapeutic devices. The scientists reasoned that the lack of evidence of the fish oils was due to the low overall occurrence of events[584].
- 87 patients with coronary artery disease were supplemented with 1. 65g of omega-3 and compared to 84 control patients and global numbers for two years. The results showed a nonsignificant increase in intima-media thickness in the omega-3 group as measured by ultrasound[585].
- In 2005, 200 patients with a recent episode of ventricular failure of ventricular tachycardia and an implantable defibrillator were segregated into a +/- 1.3-gram fish oil per

day group or a placebo. Both ventricle failure and ventricle tachycardia events were significantly higher in the fish oil group[586].

- In 1995, results were published after collecting data from 14,916 patients. Each patient with an infarction was compared with a participant without an infarction. After five years, results showed a non-significant trend towards an increase in infarctions among higher fish oil levels[587].

- In 2009, 102 patients with confirmed stroke were divided into 1 group of fish oil and 1 group of palm-soy oil combination. After 12 weeks, there was no difference in health parameters (LDL, triglycerides, inflammatory and hemostatic properties) and mood. However, there was a massive increase in peroxidation levels between pre- and post-treatment after fish oil supplementation at a rate of at least 400%[588].

- In Finland, a study was financed to investigate the effects of mercury and fish oil's effects on a stroke. The study followed over 1800 people for more than 20 years. The study found a significant positive association between slightly higher mercury levels and high levels of fish oil and increased amounts of strokes[589].

Cardiac Health

An irregular heartbeat (arrhythmia) can cause cardiac death. In 2012 it was observed that pre-treated dogs with a fish oil intake of 1-4 grams per day not only failed to prevent arrhythmia but produced ventricular fibrillation in 33% of dogs (versus 0% of placebo) that were previously resistant to ventricular fibrillation, leaving the scientist to conclude reconsidering including fish oil post-myocardial infarction patients[590]. In 2012, 2 groups of sheep (fish oil and placebo) were each stressed with doxorubicin - a chemotherapy drug that is known to cause heart failure and is toxic to the heart. It was found that the fish oil group showed an increase in left ventricle dilation and reduced output of oxygen-rich blood into the bloodstream (decline in ejection fraction)[591], which is linked to heart failure.

In 1972, they were comparing patients with heart infarctions versus healthy subjects it was found that patients had higher DHA and EPA values after evaluating the fatty acid composition in cholesterol esters, phospholipids, and triglycerides in serum[592]. Studies comparing saturated fats and polyunsaturated fats regarding heart health show some impressive results. In 2012, Galvao found that saturated fat increased heart failure survival rate in hamsters when compared to unsaturated (omega-3 and 6) or low-fat diet, despite mitochondria defects[593]. One year later, the same group saw no improvement in survival rates when only omega-3 was supplied[594]. With arrhythmias, many studies with humans found that omega-3 did not offer protection[595][596][597].

Heartbeat

The heart pumps the blood by contracting muscles and by electronic signals. This contraction of the heart muscle cells is the nonmodal myocyte that contracts mostly by calcium and depolarization of the potentials of a cell. The regular order of signals in different phases sets the stage for a regular heartbeat. Any disruption of this process can lead to arrhythmia. To have regular and proper signal distribution, action potentials of nonmodal myocytes usually follow five different phases. These 5 phases are thought to be mainly controlled by the various pumps and channels that push or let minerals in and out of the cell.

action potential

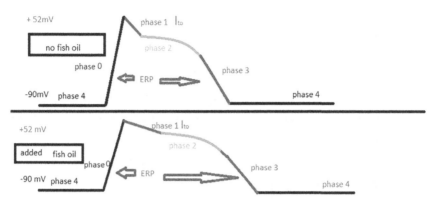

Many anti-arrhythmic drugs target the different channels to make phases longer to increase the duration of the action potential; this increases the effective refractory period (ERP), which decreases one's heartbeat per minute. Fish oil has been found to inhibit many phases, but especially in phase 1 (Ito). This is the phase that increases potassium into the cell, causing a dip in voltage (as is shown above). One of the problems with fish oils is that they have many opposing functions by blocking different channels making consistent findings difficult[598]. Different animals have different effects and even within one species, such as humans:

"These species variations serve as a cautionary note about generalizing animal studies to the clinical situation. They also suggest that the effects of FO supplementation on the cardiac electrical activity in people can vary due

to differences in genetic makeup and conditions of the heart"[599]

Xu X, Jiang M, Wang Y, Smith T, Baumgarten CM, Wood MA, et al. (2010) Long-Term Fish Oil Supplementation Induces Cardiac Electrical Remodeling by Changing Channel Protein Expression in the Rabbit Model. PLoS ONE 5(4): e10140. https://doi.org/10.1371/journal.pone.0010140

Fish-Free Diet

Patients with phenylketonuria (an inherited disease characterized by the absence or deficiency of the enzyme phenylalanine hydroxylase), can quickly build up amino acid phenylalanine to dangerous levels. The treatment for phenylketonuria is to limit these amino acids. For these patients, animal protein sources are limited, and fish is often restricted, leading to a "deficiency" in EPA and DHA via the diet. These patients have to rely on desaturase and elongase enzymes. These patients have no early signs of atherosclerotic changes and enhanced platelet activation on a fish-free diet. Furthermore, the EPA and the DHA blood levels of these patients are within the normal range[600].

Creating A Dangerous Environment

The chylomicrons that carry fish oil into the bloodstream from the lymphatic vessels can oxidize and become cytotoxic. In contrast, monounsaturated or saturated fat show no or minimal toxicity[601]. The initial lesion that can form a hazardous plaque is probably created by some injury to the vascular wall, which attracts macrophages leading to foam cells. Compared to the normal intima (inner lining of the vessel), macrophages within the lesions contain significant amounts of 7β-hydroxycholesterol. 7β-hydroxycholesterol can be easily formed after cholesterol comes in contact with unsaturated fats. It has been noted that 7β-hydroxycholesterol is rapidly created after fish oil supplementation[602]. Macrophages containing fish oil have an increased potential to oxidize LDL, even when compared to corn oil[603]. Oxidized LDL is associated with plaque instability[604].

Lipid peroxidation (including fish oil breakdown products) is an increase in diabetes[605]. In 2003 it was shown that in diabetic patients, fish oils increase the susceptibility of LDL oxidation and have pro-atherosclerosis activities[606]. This came after the results of a 1994 study that LDL increased with fish oils and showed a distinct pattern of volatile oxidation products[607]. LDL was found to increase oxidation after fish oils in many studies[608][609]. When rats are fed solely fish oils in the diet, both cholesterol and triglycerides are depressed, compared to rats who are fed soybean oil. The fish oil-fed rats, however, develop fatty streaks in the aorta and have increased ductular cell hyperplasia (overgrowth of cells that line the small ducts) in their livers[610]. In 1998, it was shown that fish oils are toxic to the livers of rabbits[611]. When large amounts of vitamin E are added to the diet, the toxicity was significantly reduced, but still present[612].

Rats' hearts were compared after two months on corn oil or salmon oil diet (and a low-fat diet). They found it that the hearts in the salmon-fed group had a mild accumulation of the ventricular chamber of lipofuscin-like material[613]. Coconut oil, olive oil, and fish oils were fed to rats for 16 weeks. It was concluded that coconut oils showed the least amount of oxidized protein and peroxidized lipids. In contrast, fish oils showed the highest amount of oxidative stress in cardiac mitochondria. The authors of the study concluded that a diet enriched with saturated fat offers powerful advantages[614].

"These data indicate that although long-term fish oil supplementation may be beneficial in reducing plasma total TG, susceptibility of plasma lipids to free radical attack is potentiated."[615]

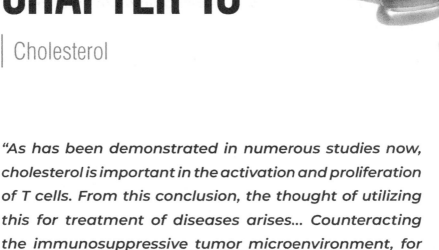

CHAPTER 10

"As has been demonstrated in numerous studies now, cholesterol is important in the activation and proliferation of T cells. From this conclusion, the thought of utilizing this for treatment of diseases arises... Counteracting the immunosuppressive tumor microenvironment, for example, could be an important aspect of all cancer therapies, potentially raising their chances of success across the board"[616]

Bietz A, Zhu H, Xue M and Xu C (2017) Cholesterol Metabolism in T Cells. Front. Immunol. 8:1664. doi: 10.3389/fimmu.2017.01664

"In conclusion, decreasing cholesterol levels or persistently low cholesterol levels were associated with higher risk of all-cause, cancer and CVD mortality. In addition, increasing cholesterol levels or persistently high cholesterol levels was also associated with high CVD mortality risk. This suggests that decreased cholesterol and low cholesterol levels may be an indicator for poor health status. The clinical implication of this study is that

individuals with spontaneously decreased cholesterol or persistently low cholesterol levels are at increased risk of mortality and may require careful attention for signs of deterioration of health" [617]

Jeong S-M, Choi S, Kim K, Kim S-M, Lee G, Son JS, et al. (2018) Association of change in total cholesterol level with mortality: A population-based study. PLoS ONE 13(4): e0196030. https://doi.org/10.1371/journal.pone.0196030

The main reason fish oil was pushed as a health supplement was under the auspices of its ability to lower cholesterol. Outperforming the fish oil theory in its duration, and probably in its fragility, the cholesterol history is worth mentioning. I am not suggesting that high cholesterol is a good thing (high cholesterol could mean a low thyroid function). I simply think that lowering cholesterol by taking PUFA is not necessarily a useful act.

Low LDL High HDL

Low cholesterol comprising of a high HDL and low LDL cholesterol ratio has been the mantra for a healthy heart for the last 60 years. HDL is high-density lipoprotein and carries cholesterol to the liver to be excreted. In contrast, low-density lipoprotein brings cholesterol to the cell from the liver. There are four types of lipoproteins (HDL, LDL, chylomicron, and VLDL) that transports fatty acids (TAG) and cholesterol through the bloodstream and lymph system. Most governmental agencies and science councils promote the idea that saturated fats increase cholesterol and thereby increase coronary artery disease (CAD). The USDA/USDHHS, the Institute of Medicine and the European Food Safety Authority have the same general recommendations: to limit consumption of saturated fat and replace it with PUFA/MUFA or carbohydrates. These recommendations are based on a meta-analysis that left out studies that show alternative outcomes or include multiple studies from the same data set, making it appear more convincing[618]. In 1982, the National Research Council warned about the effects of low cholesterol by way of unsaturated fats by increasing cancer, as many studies showed an increase of tumors associated with low cholesterol[619]. Tumor growth was seen particularly when total fat intake was low. The mono-unsaturated and saturated fats were seen as protective against the poly-unsaturated fats.

21st-Century Research

The 21st century was not a good time for the cholesterol theory. In 2000, it was shown that high HDL was associated with premature death[620], and a review of studies showed that above 60 years of age, most people showed an inverse association of high LDL with mortality[621]. It also showed that people with an inherited mutation resulting in higher HDL levels had a higher risk for coronary heart disease[622], and increased risk of ischemic heart disease for specific groups[623]. In 2002, heart failure mortality was found to be strongly associated with low cholesterol and low LDL levels[624]. In Italy, it was confirmed that higher total cholesterol was found to be very protective of brain health. After reviewing more than 4000 older people, the researchers advised physicians to see lower cholesterol as a warning sign[625]. In 2008, high cholesterol was found to be associated with better memory function[626]. In Brazil, in 2011, after following 800 people aged 65-80 for 12 years, results showed that high total cholesterol and LDL were not associated with mortality, but low total cholesterol was associated with high mortality[627]. The same results were seen after following 700 older people for six years, and it was shown that low cholesterol levels had higher levels of death independent of health status[628]. After following 1167 subjects with chronic hemodialysis for ten years, it was demonstrated that hypocholesterolemia (low cholesterol) was an independent risk factor, while 200-219 mg/dl, which is seen as high, was the most protective[629]. Published in 2013, with following more than 12,000 healthy subjects for up to 11 years, it was found that high cholesterol was protective against overall mortality, while low cholesterol was found to have increased mortality[630]. In 2008, after examining 2500 older people, it was found that the low cholesterol group resulted in a twofold increased risk of dying compared to the high cholesterol group[631]. In 2017 it was noted that men with high cholesterol had better sperm quality[632]. In the Czech Republic, women with the highest cholesterol levels were found to have the highest chance of in-hospital mortality. In contrast, those with the lowest cholesterol levels had the highest death rate after 78 months, suggesting an association factor instead of causative[633]. Beyond low cholesterol, low LDL can be very harmful. Low LDL is associated with osteoporosis in diabetic patients[634]. A systematic review for hemorrhage strokes found that among 23 studies, with a total of 1.4 million participants, high cholesterol levels and high LDL decreased the change of having hemorrhage strokes[635].

Cholesterol Degradation

Apolipoprotein is a protein that is made in the liver and can bind to fats and cholesterol to carry through the lymph and circulatory system. ApoB100 is very important for the formation of triglycerides and is the main protein in LDL. One of the ways how fish oil lowers cholesterol is the degradation of apoB100 in the liver. The way this can happen is due to lipid peroxidation that occurs in the liver. The lipid peroxidation, especially aldehydes, cross-link with proteins and the lipoprotein and is targeted for degradation[636]. The way by which fish oil lowers apoB100 is not healthy.

In comparison, the thyroid, for example, will also lower apoB100. The thyroid can reduce apoB100 by reducing the production of apoB100 in the liver, which is less toxic[637]. Thyroid hormone can reduce LDL to convert LDL cholesterol into protective properties like pregnenolone, progesterone, DHEA, and testosterone.

History Of Cholesterol And Heart Disease

The foundation of the cholesterol-heart disease theory started in Russia in 1913 when cholesterol and vegetable oil (sunflower) was added to the diet of rabbits, and atherosclerosis then occurred[638].

Many accounts were written arguing against the cholesterol theory. Already in 1926, it was found that:

- Giving rabbits "small" 25mlg amounts of cholesterol per day did not contribute to atherosclerosis. This small amount, however, 25mlg, corresponds to 750 mg per day for humans, and the daily intake for humans is recommended at 300 mg per day.
- When rabbits were fed 113 mg per day for a long duration (300+ days), only 1 out of 19 rabbits had atherosclerosis (113mlg per day would correspond to about 3390 mg cholesterol per day). The one rabbit that had atherosclerosis had normal cholesterol blood levels.

- Only when 25 rabbits were fed 253.65 mg per day did atherosclerosis occur in 9 of the subjects, or 36% (253.65mlg per day corresponds with 7609.5 mg per day).
- When 507.3 mg cholesterol was given, 5 out of 7 rabbits (71%) were shown to have atherosclerosis. This resembles 15.219 mg per day - to put this into perspective, to consume this amount of cholesterol in food, you would have to eat about 16.91 kg of steak.

The same study showed that when a high protein diet was fed to rabbits, it produced arteriosclerosis quickly. The researchers concluded that the small amount of cholesterol in the protein could not be the causative factor, but rather the high dose of protein that caused atherosclerosis and lesions[639].

In 1939, it was found that rabbits respond differently to cholesterol than other mammals do. While rabbits reacted in a heart unhealthy way, rats and guinea pigs fed more cholesterol per body weight showed no atherosclerosis. It was concluded that atheroma is not the only outcome of high cholesterol levels in the blood[640]. When rabbits were given a thyroid supplement at the same time as the cholesterol feeding, no atherosclerosis deposits were found[641]. High cholesterol levels were often known at this time to be a sign of hypothyroidism. A thyroid supplement consistently could bring cholesterol levels down (thyroid and vitamin A are needed for the conversion of cholesterol into the steroid hormones).

The Keys Studies

Before the Ancel Keys published his findings, which showed that selected countries demonstrated an association between fat, cholesterol, and heart disease, the idea of cholesterol as the primary cause was ridiculed. One scientist wrote that cholesterol advocates have to go through "mental gymnastics" to try to prove their point[642].

At the time that Keys published his cholesterol data of 1492 Minnesota students, the mean cholesterol was low compared to Illinois and British students, Danish hospital employees, and factory workers. In the 1950s, scientists wondered whether Keys students had characteristics that would provide lower levels of cholesterol. One scientist argued that the multitude of students of Scandinavian descent among Keys' subjects skewed the results. Furthermore, cold weather increases cholesterol, and Minnesota is one of the coldest states in the USA.

Other Historical Cholesterol Studies

The case against the causative role of cholesterol grew when studies started to show that groups with different cholesterol levels had similar survival rates[643644]. One group of scientists reasoned that cholesterol was picked due to the ease at which it could be measured - they presumed that cholesterol was getting too much attention and found no basis that heart disease is due to a deficiency in PUFA[645]. At that same time, it was observed that as we age, our metabolic rate decreases, and that this decrease is associated with atherosclerosis[646]. It was shown that cholesterol could cause atherosclerosis when dogs were given thyroid suppressors[647]. In the 1950s, significant observations were made that should have put cholesterol in a different perspective. Cholesterol was found to keep steadily rising in both males and females. Until in men up to about age 50, the cholesterol levels stop increasing, while in women, cholesterol kept rising until a later age. At the time, it was known that women lived longer than men. This fact has been confirmed in another study[648]. Furthermore, it was observed that low cholesterol was present in infections, anemia, sprue, leprosy, and kala-azar[649].

Furthering Keys' Work

At about the same time as Keys was conducting his studies in the early 1950s, in the north of Europe, other findings were published. In Denmark, Gaviand found an association between lipid peroxides and the degree of atherosclerosis. In contrast, in normal aortas, no lipid peroxides were found[650]. Although many voices were arguing against the cholesterol theory, Sinclair furthered Keys' work and published in 1956 in The Lancet a hypothesis that the saturated fatty esters of cholesterol caused atherosclerosis degeneration together with a deficiency in the essential fatty acids.

Sinclair urged scientists to test this hypothesis, and this challenge was taken up by the Dutch chemist C.J.F. Böttcher. To Böttcher's surprise, the arterial plaques consisted of a high volume of the unsaturated fatty acids, and the more advanced atherosclerotic plaques contained more linoleic and arachidonic acid (omega-6).

In C.J.F. Böttcher's memoirs, he comments that this news was not pleasantly received by the Dutch conglomerate Unilever (who commercialized margarine). When Böttcher went to the United States, he found that the reason he had received a harsh treatment was because the wealthy medical professionals had their fortunes invested in the newly planted crops used for unsaturated fats[651]. Böttcher wrote that scientists sometimes favored greed over science.

Böttcher kept working on atherosclerosis and concluded that atherosclerosis is a disease of the arterial intima in its entirety, even in areas of apparent structural normality[652]. Böttcher called the role of cholesterol in regards to atherosclerosis "modest". These and other studies led the Learned Society of the Netherlands to conclude that blood cholesterol is less important than was speculated initially[653]. From 1955 to 1960, many councils and authors warned against the cholesterol theory and the marketing efforts surrounding unsaturated fats and ways to lower cholesterol[654655].

Metabolic Rate

Research continued along the lines of oxygen uptake and metabolic rate. As organisms age, their oxygen uptake and metabolic rate decrease. Careful experiments have shown that the decreased metabolic rate often leads to reduced integrity of vessels and other organs. Decreased integration of the endothelium leads to the accumulation of cholesterol versus intact tissue (which again suggests that cholesterol is an aid to injured tissue)[656].

In 1965, the Japanese scientist Iwakami was thinking along the same lines but included the breakdown products of unsaturated fats (peroxides). Iwakami knew that peroxides inhibit necessary oxidative enzymes and reduce the production of ATP (energy). This reduction in energy leads to an inability to function normally. Iwakami thought that peroxides were the primary cause of arteriosclerosis inhibition of oxidative enzymes[657]. It was found that the area with the highest arteriosclerosis (aortic arch) showed high oxygen consumption, letting the scientist of the day think that this was a sign of "increased energy requirement"[658].

Iwakami and Gaviand were ahead of their time - scientists at the time did not think in terms of peroxides and unsaturated fats and health. Lipid peroxidation research was confined to laboratory research. Only 20 years later did scientists think that lipid peroxidation could have an impact on health. Since the late 1980s, research has proven that lipid peroxidation is implicated in many diseases[659].

"Until the '80s, lipid peroxidation was confined to specialized laboratories in which the phenomenon was mainly evaluated in vitro. At this stage, researchers were interested in reproducing lipid peroxidation as a macrophenomenon induced by xenobiotics of such an entity that would be quite unlikely to be present in human physiology and pathology."[660]

Signorini C, De Felice C, Durand T, et al. Isoprostanes and 4-hydroxy-2-nonenal: markers or mediators of disease? Focus on Rett syndrome as a model of autism spectrum disorder. Oxid Med Cell Longev. 2013;2013:343824. doi:10.1155/2013/343824

Despite many studies showing that cholesterol was not necessarily the culprit in heart disease, the trend was set and thus continued. Recent discoveries have shown that carefully conducted studies from the 1960s and 1970s showed that vegetable oils were proven to be potentially very harmful.

- After Keys showed that high cholesterol was associated with ischaemic heart disease, a research team divided 80 patients randomly into 1 of 3 groups. Group 1 was the control group, to which no advice was given. Group 2 was assigned 80 grams of olive oil a day, while group 3 was fed the experimental corn oil (80 grams per day). Both the olive and corn group were advised to avoid saturated fats and animal products. Although the study was planned for three years, the results were published after two years. Cholesterol did go down in the corn oil group; however, the number of deaths went up. After two years, the data were graded according to the patients' status of remaining alive and free of re-infarction. The control group had 75% alive and well, the olive oil had 57% alive and well, while the corn oil group only had 52% that fared well[661].

- The Sydney Diet Study ran from 1966 till 1973, selecting 458 participants between 30 and 59 years of age-specific people with a recent coronary event. The control group (n=237) had no interventions. In contrast, the experimental group (n=221) all saturated fats were replaced with sunflower oil or sunflower margarine. The results showed that the sunflower oil group had a reduced cholesterol level, together with an increase in all causes of mortality, cardiovascular disease, and death from coronary heart disease. The experimental group reached a death rate of 17.6%, while the control group only reached an 11.8% death rate[662].

- At around the same time, from 1968-1973, the Minnesota Conorary Experiment was executed. The study included 9423 people aged 20-97. The control group's diet was high (er) in saturated fats, while in the experimental group, these fats were replaced mainly by the cholesterol-lowering corn oil fat. The data was re-evaluated in 2016, and the evaluation found a 22% higher risk of death for each 30 mg/ DL decrease in cholesterol[663].

- In 1964 a research team wanted to test the hypothesis if a deficiency of the essential fatty acids is associated with the trend of incidence of coronary heart disease. The research team collected data from 1909 onwards. The most striking trends were the increase in simple sugars and a slight increase in fat. More in-depth research found that the ratio of essential fatty acid (PUFA) to saturated fat increases to 37%, making the researcher conclude that the rise in coronary heart disease due to low essential fatty acid intake is not supported by the data[664].

The initial cholesterol study from 1913 showed that feeding cholesterol with vegetable oil caused heart disease. In 1987, scientists wanted to figure out if fish oils could reduce the feeding of cholesterol to rabbits. The rabbits were divided into three groups. Group 1 was cholesterol-free, group 2 was fed added cholesterol, group 3 was fed cholesterol plus fish oils. The results after five months showed that rabbits with cholesterol plus fish oils (group 3) had almost 60% more aortic atherosclerosis lesions than rabbits with only the added cholesterol (group 2). The scientist blamed the high amounts of malondialdehyde for the increase in lesions[665].

"total cholesterol level lower than 160 mg/dL was common in patients with acute ICH and was associated with greater neurological severity on presentation and poor 3-month outcomes"[666] ICH =intracerebral hemorrhage

Chen Y-W, Li C-H, Yang C-D, Liu C-H, Chen C-H, Sheu J-J, et al. (2017) Low cholesterol level associated with severity and outcome of spontaneous intracerebral hemorrhage: Results from Taiwan Stroke Registry. PLoS ONE 12 (4): e0171379. https://doi.org/10.1371/journal.pone.0171379

CHAPTER 11

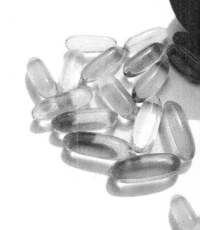

Omega-3, It's A No-Brainer

"Our results give some support to the hypothesis that high fish consumption protects against depression. This holds true for the men but not for the women. However, there were no clear associations between omega-3 PUFAs and the occurrence of depressive episodes. Therefore, the beneficial effect in the men may derive from other nutritional compounds than omega-3 PUFAs such as high quality protein, vitamins or minerals"[667]

Suominen-Taipale AL, Partonen T, Turunen AW, Männistö S, Jula A, Verkasalo PK (2010) Fish Consumption and Omega-3 Polyunsaturated Fatty Acids in Relation to Depressive Episodes: A Cross-Sectional Analysis. PLoS ONE 5 (5): e10530. https://doi.org/10.1371/journal.pone.0010530

Fish oils are supposed to make you smarter. They are thought to be particularly necessary for young children for their growing brains. The newest trend in children's candy consists of adding DHA and EPA, which is sold at room temperature sold at stores. Flavors are combined to mask the smell, making it impossible for consumers to taste the state of the oils. The brain is a unique organ that is thought to have almost exclusively postmitotic cells. The brain is usually only about 2% of body weight, but it consumes 20% of body oxygen. The iron content and high metabolic rate and temperature make it a dangerous place for unsaturated fats to exist.

"The brain is particularly vulnerable because of its high oxygen consumption and hence generation of ROS combined with a high PUFA content and modest antioxidant defences"[668]

Assies J, Pouwer F, Lok A, Mocking RJT, Bockting CLH, Visser I, et al. (2010) Plasma and Erythrocyte Fatty Acid Patterns in Patients with Recurrent Depression: A Matched Case-Control Study. PLoS ONE 5 (5): e10635. https://doi. org/10.1371/journal.pone.0010635

The brain consists roughly between 60% white matter and 40% gray matter. The gray matter has more DHA content (30-40%) than white matter (4%)[669]. The gray matter seems more susceptible than white matter, and DHA could be about 2.5 times more sensitive to oxidize than AA (omega-6). There is a significant trend of adding omega-3 to baby formula. The quantity of DHA in breast milk is reflective of the diet, and fats are predominantly stored in the brain and central nervous system. It has been found that the nervous system contains about 1/3 of the total fatty acids in the DHA form. The brain can incorporate DHA from ALA and readily does.

Brain research, IQ, genes, and eugenics are very much intertwined, from a historical perspective. Combined with the many nutrients that people lacked in the past made many scientists think in terms of deficiencies instead of excesses. Below are some examples as to why lipid peroxidation and the enzymatic products from fish oil can be dangerous for the brain.

The anterior cingulate cortex (ACC) is seen as a unique and essential part of the brain as it is a bridge between the old limbic system and the more newly formed cognitive prefrontal cortex. In the brains of deceased Alzheimer's patients compared to a control group, the Alzheimer's brain has an increase of 33% of PUFA in the ACC, including a 73% increase of DHA, resulting in a 44% increase in peroxability[670].

Prion disease

Prions are proteins that can change other proteins abnormally. It is thought that the conversion of the prion PrPc into PrPSc has a central pathology in prion disease. As it was hypothesized that cholesterol reduction would benefit the condition, both DHA and EPA and prion-infected neuron cells were experimented with. The results showed in fish-oil-treated cell lines that cholesterol was reduced, but PrPSc was doubled compared to the control[671]. Neuron cells pre-treated with DHA and EPA and incubated with a part of the prion protein have an increased chance of death[672]. The authors of the study suggest that PUFA supplements might speed up neural cell loss in Alzheimer's disease (AD).

Alpha-synuclein

Alpha-synuclein is a protein inside of the cell that has an unknown function in the healthy brain but is heavily associated with Parkinson's disease. Synuclein is found in the lipofuscin (almost exclusively) in the lower brainstem nuclei in AD[673]. Alpha-synuclein has a preference to be associated with PUFA versus saturated fats[674] and increases its pathological effects. DHA increases α-synuclein and its gene expressions[675]. Inside the cytoplasm, long-term DHA aids alpha-synuclein transformation in amyloid-like fibrils[676]. Recent studies postulated the idea of alpha-synuclein as a possible healthy feature that protects against the adverse effects of DHA operating as vitamin E acting as a lipid peroxide quencher[677].

Specialized Diets and DHA

Patients with Alzheimer's disease often have other issues like intestinal diseases and require specialized diets. One of those diets is based on peptamen, which is reportedly easily absorbed. When mice are placed on peptamen and DHA, amyloid production was increased[678].

In aging models in mice, it was observed that both EPA and DHA are both toxic to the brain as they increase BAX (BAX is a gene that can start the process of cell death). Even though the fish oil decreased omega-6 end products, scientists warned to re-evaluate the safety of EPA and DHA and concluded that both DHA and EPA "have toxic effects"[679].

DHA can replace omega-6, which was associated with severe brain swelling (encephalopathy). It has been well established that PUFA, especially omega-6 (but also omega-3), causes edema more often compared to saturated and mono-unsaturated fat[680]. One of the lipid peroxidation products from fish oils (protein-bound acrolein) is a powerful marker for Alzheimer's and was not seen in control groups[681].

Fish oils are known to increase the leaking or oozing of liquid, which is known as exudative diathesis. While it was found that the linoleic series (omega-6) tended to cause encephalomalacia (omega-3 can also cause 'crazy chick disease'), the linolenic series (omega-3) tend to cause exudative diathesis in vitamin E deficient animals. The chicks developed exudative diathesis as early as the 9th day of the experiment when fed the ethyl esters or reconstituted triglycerides obtained from the most unsaturated fractions of fish oil. The observed disorders are not due to the ethyl ester form of the fatty acids or to the oxidation of the oil in the feed[682].

When looking at the symptoms of exudative diathesis, one can see the potential dangers of omega-3 supplementations. Exudative refers to the fluid that enters (oozes) into lesions or specific sites from the circulatory systems. At the same time, diathesis is defined as a tendency to suffer from a particular medical condition. This oozing of fluid was recently clearly demonstrated when rats were fed fish oils to see the effects after surgery on short- and long-term behavior. The results, however, showed an increase in reperfusion-related hemorrhage: 37.9% in the omega-3 groups vs. 0% in the basal group. These unexpected results resulted in increased deaths, which left the researchers unable to conduct any further experiments[683] (see graph below). The decrease of energy and proneness to oxidize makes the cell less stable, and fluid can leak from the cells and plasma through membranes to the extracellular fluid, causing edema.

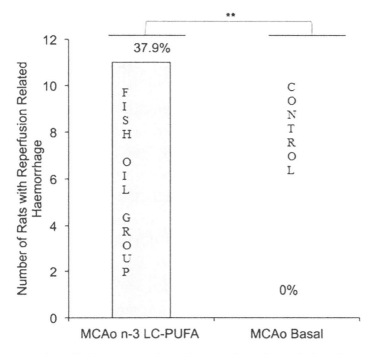

Number of MCAo operated rats that experienced reperfusion related hemorrhage, between diet conditions. MCAo, middle cerebral artery occlusion surgery condition; Basal, basal diet fed rats; n-3-LC-PUFA, polyunsaturated fatty acid supplemented rats; n = 11 n-3-LC-PUFA MCAo; n = 0 basal MCAo

Elinder F and Liin SI (2017) Actions and Mechanisms of Polyunsaturated Fatty Acids on Voltage-Gated Ion Channels. Front. Physiol. 8:43. doi: 10.3389/fphys.2017.00043

"Therefore, some authors argue that it is prudent to ensure that patients who are classified as high risk for hemorrhage discontinue n-3-LC-PUFA consumption"[684]

Pascoe MC, Howells DW, Crewther DP, Constantinou N, Carey LM, Rewell SS, Turchini GM, Kaur G and Crewther SG (2014) Fish oil diet associated with acute reperfusion related hemorrhage, and with reduced stroke-related sickness behaviors and motor impairment. Front. Neurol. 5:14. doi: 10.3389/fneur.2014.00014

The aforementioned trans-4-hydroxy-2-hexenal (HHE), an aldehyde derived from DHA, was found to be toxic to primary cultures of cerebral cortical neurons with about the same lethality as the omega-6 isomer (from AA). The amount of DHA in the brain is 30-50% higher than the AA, making it potentially much more dangerous[685]. Compared to controls, patients with mild cognitive impairment (MCI) have an increase in F(4)-NP (F(4)-neuroprostane (F(4)-NP). F(4)-NP in the brain can be derived from DHA. The only difference between MCI and late AD was significantly increased F4-NP in the hippocampus in advanced AD[686]. After these observations, the scientist deduced that oxidative damage might be implicated at the beginning of Alzheimer's disease. The onset of brain diseases is associated with mitochondria dysfunction[687]. Mitochondria susceptibility to damage is increased when the mitochondrial membrane is increased with omega-3, compared to beef tallow[688].

When Alzheimer's patients are compared to ordinary people in different brain regions (middle frontal and inferior temporal gyri and cerebellum), it was shown that DHA is the only fat (out of 6) that has higher values in Alzheimer's patients[689]. DHA increases from healthy persons to asymptomatic Alzheimer's disease patients to post mortem bodies with significant AD. *The scientist mentioned using "great caution" when using fish oil supplementation in neurological conditions after it was found that omega-3 has the potential to worsen the prognosis of ALS by increasing 4-hydroxy-2-hexenal. The authors wrote:*

"These data show that dietary EPA supplementation in ALS has the potential to worsen the condition and accelerate the disease progression."[690]

Yip PK, Pizzasegola C, Gladman S, Biggio ML, Marino M, Jayasinghe M, et al. (2013) The Omega-3 Fatty Acid Eicosapentaenoic Acid Accelerates Disease Progression in a Model of Amyotrophic Lateral Sclerosis. PLoS ONE 8 (4): e61626. https://doi.org/10.1371/journal.pone.0061626

While the influx of the omega-6 levels seems to be regulated in the brain and controlled, omega-3 fatty acids do not seem to have these mechanisms. When mice are fed 17% instead of 2.2% omega-6, brain levels remain constant. When cod liver oil or salmon oil is added at concentrations of 14.5% or 12.5%, respectively, brain levels are increased in favor of omega-3, leaving scientists to caution about the excessive intake of omega-3, because it would be difficult to reverse[691]. Below is an observation that is often observed in studies with depressed patients, that the total PUFA is higher than controls.

"The Σ ω-6 PUFAs in plasma was significantly higher in the patients than in the controls consistent with a higher intake of mainly LA. However, in contrast to many earlier studies, we found that levels of AA, EPA, DHA and the Σ ω-3 PUFAs in plasma were similar in patients and controls, as were AA/EPA and AA/DHA ratios"[692]

Assies J, Pouwer F, Lok A, Mocking RJT, Bockting CLH, Visser I, et al. (2010) Plasma and Erythrocyte Fatty Acid Patterns in Patients with Recurrent Depression: A Matched Case-Control Study. PLoS ONE 5 (5): e10635. https://doi.org/10.1371/journal.pone.0010635

Infants And Fish Oils

One of the fastest-growing sectors of fish oil revenue is the adding of DHA and EPA to infant formula. Adding oils in infant formula has been done in the past, mostly for premature infants. While adding extra proteins can cause excess fluid in the body, and infants do not have a lot of enzymes to digest carbohydrates. Oils, therefore, are considered an excellent addition to providing extra calories for premature infants. Although adding oils was initially started to add calories for growth, it has transformed into adding "essential fats," including DHA in the formula. One study from India found that coconut oil outperformed safflower oil for premature infants. The authors of the study cautioned against routine, adding fats and suggested an individualistic approach to adding oil. They stated, about oil fortification in infant formula:

"The technique of oil fortification is fraught with dangers of intolerance, contamination and aspiration. Long-term effects of such supplementation are largely unknown"[693]

Vaidya UV, Hegde VM, Bhave SA, Pandit AN. Vegetable oil fortified feeds in the nutrition of very low birthweight babies. Indian Pediatr. 1992;29(12):1519–1527.

Very early in food research, Pappenheimer showed that vitamin E deficiency caused no or little effect on the pregnant mother. Still, adverse effects could be seen in the offspring. A little later, it was observed that a vitamin E deficiency could prolong pregnancy. This is relevant as fish oil, which can induce vitamin E deficiency, is often given to pregnant mothers to prolong pregnancy. This perceived advantage was found to be a disadvantage after an increase in EPA was associated with a decrease in "birthweight adjusted for gestational age"[694]. Furthermore, fish oil decrease PGE2, which is a potent labor inducer. The importance of omega-3 is usually seen as there is a considerable increase of DHA in the third trimester in the infant's brain. This increase of DHA, in particular, is associated with brain growth and health. A more logical line of reasoning would be that the rise of estrogen in the third trimester needed to induce labor. The decrease in progesterone and testosterone would increase the unsaturation of unsaturated fats, leaving the increase in unsaturation (mostly omega-6), a contributor to induce labor[695][696].

It is important to note that breast milk, although dependent on the mother's diet, is usually very low in these unsaturated fatty acids. DHA, for example, is only 0.3% of content by weight[697]. Furthermore, animal experiments show that the offspring has mechanisms in place for long periods without DHA[698]. The proteins in breast milk are very protective against lipid peroxidation (especially casein)[699]. The DHA and other longer unsaturated fatty acids decrease while saturated fats increase during breastfeeding[700]. With DHA, more is not better. In 1987 it was found that 11mg/kg/day, given at different times, absorbed more or equal amounts of DHA compared to 71mg/kg/day[701]. Lower intake of DHA does not result in lower intellectual development. One study compared low DHA formula infants versus breastfed infants and found their development to be the same as two years of age[702].

| IQ

As with many omega-3 research studies, the substitution of omega-3 with fish consumption is often made. When the association between high fish intake and higher IQ in the offspring is made, many articles appear stating increase omega-3 intakes will likely lead to higher IQ, thereby excluding all other possible favorable molecules present, and forgetting its possible worse substitutes[703]. Despite the outward public view that omega-3 can do no wrong, controversy exists about supplementing with these fragile fats for the developing child. Let us have a look at some of these studies.

- In 1992 a study found that marine oil (omega-3) fed infants had poorer scores regarding weight, length, and head circumferences[704].
- A Dutch study found that the infants of mothers receiving DHA had a more inferior quality general movement. Furthermore, the DHA had almost double the mildly abnormal general movements compared to other groups[705].
- In 2012 results were published following three groups of infants: the first group received omega-3 and omega-6 supplementation (DHA at 0.30% body weight, AA omega-6, 0.45% body weight) for two months; the second group received the standard infant formula and functioned as a control group, and in the third group infants were breastfed. The results showed that at age 9, the breastfed fared best, while the infant formula group without the added DHA and AA compared to the added oil group did better in cognitive functions than the experimental group from non-smoking mothers (the researchers blamed attrition)[706].
- Infants were again divided into three groups (DHA supplemented, DHA plus omega-6, and infant supplement without long-chain fatty acids). These three groups were then compared with breastfed infants (a reference group). The results showed that there were no differences between the 3 groups, but found that the breastfed group had better visual evoked potential at 34 weeks and better mental development at two years of age[707].
- Between 2005 and 2009, 2399 pregnant mothers with depression from Australia were divided into a fish oil group (DHA 800 mg + EPA 100 mg daily) and a vegetable oil group (mix of rapeseed palm and sunflower daily). The infants were then followed for 18 months. Results showed fewer

children in the DHA group with scores indicating delayed cognitive development compared to the vegetable oil group. Further findings showed that girls in the DHA group had weaker adaptive behavior skills, reduced language scores compared to girls from the vegetable oil group, as well as an increased risk of delayed language improvements[708].

- In 1998, 4 groups were compared (standard formula, a formula that had been supplemented with DHA from fish oil, DHA and arachidonic acid, and a nonrandomized human milk comparison group). The researchers found that the DHA group (omega-3) scored lower on the Vocabulary Comprehension Scale and the Vocabulary Production Scale and found significant negative correlations between DHA levels and vocabulary outcomes[709].

- In 2004, ALA (omega-3) was given to pregnant women together with linoleic acid (omega-6), versus pregnant women receiving solely linoleic acid as supplementation. Infants at 32 weeks of age showed a negative association between higher DHA concentrations and cognitive performance[710].

- Passive communication is lower at age 1 with fish oil supplementation as compared to olive oil, and word comprehension at age one was inversely associated with erythrocyte-DHA at four months[711].

- Data from Norway involving 62,099 participants showed that lean fish was the driver of association with birth size (more than fatty fish) - infant head circumference was negatively associated with the mother's intake of the a-3 fatty acid supplement[712].

- In 2015, preterm infants were divided into a high DHA supplemented group (1% of total fatty acid), and a "normal" low DHA supplemented group (0.2-0.3% of total fatty acids). They were then followed up at the age of 7. At age 7, the low DHA performed slightly better on eye tests. Furthermore, the number of children with an IQ of less than 85 was almost double in the high DHA group, and the high DHA required more operations than the control group[713].

- When pregnant women's blood levels were tested for fatty acids between 1959-1967 and their offspring was tested between 1981-1997, it was observed that the offspring whose mothers had the highest DHA levels had a 200% increase in schizophrenia spectrum disorders, no such observation was found with AA or with low DHA levels[714].

"This study adds to the growing body of evidence suggesting that prenatal DHA supplementation does not have a significant overall positive effect on global measures of infant development."[715]

Ramakrishnan U, Stinger A, DiGirolamoAM, Martorell R, Neufeld LM, Rivera JA, et al. (2015)Prenatal Docosahexaenoic Acid Supplementation and Offspring Development at 18 Months:Randomized Controlled Trial. PLoS ONE 10 (8): e0120065. doi:10.1371/journal.pone.0120065

When infants formula was compared to stored breastmilk, it was found that infant formula had almost 20 times more the levels of HHE-1 (4-hydroxyhexenal) compared to breastmilk (measured per microgram/g). The peroxidation of omega-3 was found to be higher than omega-6[716]. A Korean Study calculated that an infant only fed PUFA fortified baby foods and formula from age three months to 1 year could be exposed to a 100 times more HHE and HNE than adults, per body weight per day[717].

Animal Studies

Animal studies are useful but can be challenging to interpret. As we saw with the original rabbit and cholesterol study, study results and interpretations can have enormous consequences. Even though in animal studies, vast quantities of a supplement or medicine can be given that would not be in the range of a human dose, if the control group would be assigned the same dose of another supplement or medicine, useful remarks can be made. The following examples are a summary of animal studies with regards to the brain and fish oils:

- When mice were fed an omega-3 deficient diet for three generations, the mice showed a 53% decrease of DHA in brain tissue. These omega-3 deficient mice showed a better ability to locate platforms and had reduced pain sensitivities[718].

- In an enriched environment, three groups of mice (saturated, omega-3 and 6, and an omega-3 deficient diet) showed little or no difference[719]. In contrast, fish oil-fed mice versus palm oil-fed mice showed improvements in the fish oil group during an early age, a decline in learning in old age, and increased weight[720].

- Pups of rats fed fish oil-supplemented (plus a group fed the corn oil) diet throughout pregnancy and lactation had slower rates of growth and a delay in neurodevelopment. The rats fed the fish oil were retarded in the growth of their auditory brainstem and the time of appearance of the auditory startle reflex, not seen in the corn oil group[721].

- The auditory brainstem response (ABR) was again seen in excess of fish oil (7%) during pregnancy and lactation in the pups. The surprising aspect of this study was the control group and the omega-3 deficiency group. The control group contained 7% soy, while the omega-3 deficient diet contained 7% safflower oil. The control and the omega-3 deficient group achieved better results than the fish oil group[722].

"The presence of arachidonic acid and docosahexaenoic acid in lung triglycerides correlated with the ability of these lungs to peroxidize lipids in vitro in all species. Depletion of lung triglycerides in neonatal rats by fasting abolished this lipid peroxidizing activity"[723]

Kehrer JP, Autor AP. Relationship between fatty acids and lipid peroxidation in lungs of neonates. Biol Neonate. 1978;34(1-2):61–67. doi:10.1159/000241106

Overall, most studies show little or no benefit from omega-3 fatty acids concerning brain health for the elderly, school children, infants, and depressed individuals[724][725][726][727].

| Eyes

The suggested importance of DHA is usually made clear with the eyes; as DHA accumulates in the eyes, it has been perceived that DHA is of utmost importance for eye health. In 1992, 81 low weight infants were put on different formulas and/or breast milk (all at varying levels of omega-3). At 57 weeks, no difference was seen in various eye health tests compared to DHA and EPA group versus no DHA and EPA[728]. Studies with rats show that being on long-term fat-free diets did not result in adverse findings for the eyes[729]. The researchers suggested that the body has ways of preserving DHA. Multi-generational studies show that DHA deprivation negatively affects the eye, but could be alleviated by other nutrients - see EFAD Chapter 13. When infants fed breast milk with more DHA were compared with low content DHA formula, no DHA difference in the retina was found[730]. A positive relationship has been found between the quantity of DHA in the retina, the level of lipid peroxidation (4-hydroxyhexenal) leading "to photooxidative stress"[731]. Higher levels of retinal docosahexaenoic acid do not protect mice expressing the VPP rhodopsin mutation from retinal degeneration[732].

After a one-year-long study feeding infants three different formulas containing (1) no long polyunsaturated fatty acids, (2) added DHA and AA, or (3) increased amount of DHA, various eye tests revealed no differences. It seems that moderate to high intake of DHA does not improve eye health[733], while high DHA levels could be hazardous.

In rabbits, after injections with DHA, rapid increases in malondialdehyde are seen, followed by a rapid decline. These malondialdehydes most probably attach themselves to the elements in vitreous tissue (fluid-like gel between the lens and retina, which can result in cataracts); as malondialdehydes decrease, the amounts of cataracts increase[734].

Rabbits, like rats, can generate cataracts within two years, whereas dogs can produce them in 8 years. Comparatively, whales do not develop cataracts in 200 years of life. It was recently found that whales have high levels of sphingolipids, which are known to have more saturated fatty acids than, for example, glycerolipids. The lenses of whales were also characterized by a more ordered membrane and one of the highest concentrations of cholesterol in the lens[735]. This observation of cholesterol as an anti-inflammatory agent in the lens has been described by other scientists, akin to vitamin E, in keeping the lens clear[736]. Cholesterol can scavenge to pick up lipid peroxidation products and form stable products, instead of letting these lipid peroxides form products with DNA, protein, etc. Comparing clear lenses with lenses containing cataracts, these oxidized products combined with cholesterol forming products (7α-hydroxycholesterol, 7β-hydroxycholesterol, 5α,6α-epoxycholestanol, and 7-ketocholesterol) are easily found with lenses with cataracts but are absent in clear lenses[737]. Instead of focusing on just the omega-6 eicosanoids, but rather also including the omega-3 versions found higher omega-3 derivatives (14-HDoHE) in more severe cases of Meibomian gland (MG) dysfunction (eye condition)[738].

Logical Observations

During World War II, prisoners of war were held under the cruelest of conditions with many nutritional deficiencies. One study describes 350 prisoners of war that were held by the Japanese. After being freed four years later, cataracts were found in only 2 cases, and partial optic atrophy from malnutrition was about 20%[739]. The diet was white rice-based, with minimal supplies of vegetable and rotten animal flesh. The essential fatty acid content of these diets must have been minimum. At the end of World War II, the Japanese had been starving in tents for months, living on grass and the potato tops in the Philippines. After the Japanese finally surrendered to the Allies, little or no eye problems were found[740]. Many studies showed that although prisoners of war were on limited starvation diets for years, little or no eye problems were noted[741].

Plasmalogen

"Interestingly, an antioxidant effect has also been ascribed to plasmalogens that, like a scavenger, could protect unsaturated membrane lipids. Consequently, it is proposed that the heterogeneous presence of plasmalogens in tissues is an adaptive response to offer stability and protection against oxidative stress conditions to lipid membranes"[742]

Pradas, I, Huynh, K, Cabré R, Ayala V, Meikle PJ, Jové M and Pamplona R (2018) Lipidomics Reveals a Tissue-Specific Fingerprint. Front. Physiol. 9:1165. doi: 10.3389/fphys.2018.01165

Plasmalogen is different than other phospholipids because of the vinyl ether bond at the SN-1 position. Plasmalogen gained interest within the scientific community as levels of plasmalogen are associated with longevity.

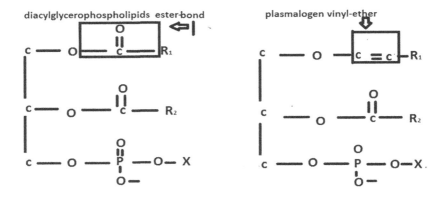

The R group (usually R2) can be an unsaturated fatty acid, and the X is a headgroup and can be part of the membrane.

A considerable amount of research has been done to decipher the role of plasmalogen. In 1924, Voight and Feulgen found that an aldehyde was attached to a substance which they named plasmalogen. In the 1950s, research began to be conducted that started to isolate the structure of plasmalogen and its lipids[743]. It was not yet possible to separate the different fats from the plasmalogen. The omega-3 family of fats seems to be more easily incorporated into plasmalogen molecules than omega-6. Plasmalogens are attacked at the SN-1 position instead of the PUFA that is likely attached to the SN-2. Because plasmalogens do not propagate like PUFA, inflammation can be significantly reduced.

How Can We Increase Plasmalogen?

In the scientific literature, one finds almost exclusively the same idea that this SN-2 position is an enrichment of the molecule. Within the culture of the "protective and deficient" fish oils, this enrichment idea makes sense. However, taking the fragile nature of the fish oil into consideration, this enrichment makes less sense. I would like to make the case that increasing fish oil in the organism decreases plasmalogen. Plasmalogen can function as a safety net for the protection of the SN-2 position. Fish oils will shorten the lifespan of plasmalogens and reduce their quantity. Because DHA can so quickly peroxidize, it can cause a loss of plasmalogen. Even compared to krill oil, which has about half the amount of DHA and EPA, plasmalogen loss was 50% in the liver compared to krill oil after fish oil or krill oil supplementation in mice[744]. When rats' testicles are examined when being fed different fatty acids consisting of different unsaturated ratios, the unsaturated fats have low plasmalogen levels; the more saturated (coconut oil and olive oil) have very high levels of plasmalogens. The same observations were seen in testosterone production and antioxidant status (higher in the more saturated group, lower in the unsaturated group)[745]. The breakdown products of fish oil (aldehydes, acrolein, etc.) can lower the plasmalogens[746]. Fish oil can lower plasmalogen levels, while plasmalogen seems to protect fish oil[747].

When rats are made deficient in PUFA, the peroxisomal fatty acid content is changed. As expected, the PUFA content of omega-3 and -6 was lowered, and the less fragile omega-9 and -7 were increased. The catalase activity is decreased (due to less need for this mechanism), and an increase in DHAPAT (dihydroxyacetone-phosphate acyltransferase) activity is noted[748]. DHAPAT is an enzyme and the initial step in the formation of plasmalogens. Decreased activity of DHAPAT leads to a reduced plasmogen production[749]. This occurs in the liver - from the liver, plasmalogen is transported by proteins into the brain and other organs. Fish oil has a well-known but not well-published relation to the liver. Fish oil can worsen many liver injuries and prevents regeneration[750][751].

Along with a healthy liver, it was found that the co-factors required for plasmalogen are CoA, ATP, Mg2+, and NADP[752]. The decrease in ATP when burning unsaturation versus glucose or even saturated fat may contribute to reducing plasmalogen production. Important locations for plasmalogen are the brain, retina, heart, and nervous system. The same sites were DHA is found. Compared to saturated fats, unsaturated fatty acids are poor substrates for DHAPAT, the best fatty acids to be used for DHAPAT for making plasmalogens seem to be 14 and 16 carbon in length (Myristic acid and Palmitic acid)[753]. In fish, there seems to be an inverse relationship between unsaturated fats and plasmalogen with regards to temperature;

as the temperature increases, unsaturated fats decrease, and plasmalogen increases[754].

Human breast milk consists primarily of long-chain fatty acids with predominantly plasmalogen in the ethanolamine form[755]. As plasmalogens offer protection against lipid peroxidation, researchers have questioned if plasmalogen could be one of the reasons that DHA in breast milk is associated with health in the infant. Plasmalogen increases just like DHA while in the womb at about 32 weeks, after which it increases in breast milk until the infant is about six months old[756]. Infant formulas typically do not contain plasmalogens[757].

CHAPTER 12

Old & New, Serotonin & Adiponectin

The next chapter focuses on molecules that are increased by omega-3 intake and have a perceived positive effect on health. The research on these molecules is still unclear, and conclusions are yet to be established. Many of these studies show an association relationship that does not prove causation. Pharmaceutical companies are at the beginning of exploiting these molecules for a variety of illnesses[758].

Adiponectin

"In Japanese men, a high adiponectin level was a risk factor for anemia. .. and our study clinically and epidemiologically shows that adiponectin negatively affects erythropoiesis"[759]

Kohno K, Narimatsu H, Shiono Y, Suzuki I, Kato Y, Sho R, et al. (2016) High Serum Adiponectin Level Is a Risk Factor for Anemia in Japanese Men: A Prospective Observational Study of 1,029 Japanese Subjects. PLoS ONE 11 (12): e0165511. https://doi.org/10.1371/journal.pone.0165511

Adiponectin is a protein hormone-like molecule secreted from adipose tissue. The ability of adiponectin to increase insulin sensitivity and its reportedly low amounts in heart patients means that it has been heavily researched. As omega-3 increases adiponectin, it is thought that one way of the potential benefits is through the fish oil adiponectin pathway[760]. In men, adiponectin has a strong inverse relationship with testosterone. When testosterone increases, adiponectin decreases, and vice versa[761]. There have been many studies showing that in old age, high adiponectin levels are something to be concerned about. Higher adiponectin levels in people with heart failure and those free of heart disease are associated with increased all-cause mortality and heart disease death[762763764765]. This relationship seems to be more than a mere association and is termed a "cause-effect relationship"[766]. Adiponectin function in part by thermo-suppression[767]. It appears to inhibit bone formation and is inversely related to bone strength[768].

Serotonin

"In fact, there is no scientifically established ideal "chemical balance" of serotonin, let alone an identifiable pathological imbalance"[769]

Lacasse JR, Leo J (2005) Serotonin and Depression: A Disconnect between the Advertisements and the Scientific Literature. PLoS Med 2(12): e392. https://doi.org/10.1371/journal.pmed.0020392

Recent developments have postulated that omega-3 and vitamin D are essential for the production of serotonin from the amino acid tryptophan. While it was found that vitamin D was involved in serotonin production, if serotonin had already been high, vitamin D would lower serotonin levels[770] (Omega-3 have not been shown to reduce serotonin levels). Omega-3 deficiency leads to lower serotonin metabolites (5-hydroxy indole acetic acid 5-HIAA), while DHA leads to higher metabolite levels. 5-HIAA is one way to measure serotonin levels. 5-HIAA levels, like the unsaturated fatty acids, are higher at night[771] . It is heavily associated with mental problems, reduced brain size, and depression, and is often increased in more severe cases[772773774775] (suicide occurrence is usually highest at night-time, with time awake adjusted[776777]).

History Of Serotonin

Serotonin has been popularized as an antidepressant working as an LSD opposer. In 1954, serotonin was seen as a healthy brain molecule as it was thought to be at low levels in patients with schizophrenia[778]. The low serotonin level theory was not proven at the time, but rather a working hypothesis.

"It must be remembered that this opinion about a cerebral serotonin deficiency as the cause of conditions such as schizophrenia is a working hypothesis. Although one can demonstrate in smooth muscles a competitive antagonism between serotonin and the various drugs just discussed, there are other explanations which can be put forward for their psychotic effects. One of these is that the mental aberrations arise from an excess of serotonin rather than from a deficiency"[779]

JOURNAL ARTICLE Some Neurophysiological Of Serotonin D. W. Woolley and E. Shaw The British Medical Journal Vol. 2, No. 4880 (Jul. 17, 1954), pp. 122-126

When injecting serotonin or precursors in laboratory animals, the results range from low doses into lethargic behavior (hibernation-like), or high doses, possibly causing effects that mimicked high doses of LSD. The scientist of the time noted that after serotonin injections, animals displayed:

"signs of clinical schizophrenia. For example, the lassitude and the willingness of the cat to remain in unnatural positions when so manoeuvred by the experimenter might be likened to the catatonia seen in some human mental disorders"[780]

JOURNAL ARTICLE Some Neurophysiological Of Serotonin D. W. Woolley and E. Shaw The British Medical Journal Vol. 2, No. 4880 (Jul. 17, 1954), pp. 122-126

Zero Energy

At around the same time that serotonin was postulated as a brain health molecule, it was found that serotonin inhibited the function of mitochondria and caused a decrease in energy. The scientist warned that serotonin could lessen brain function as it decreased phosphorus and oxygen uptake[781]. A little later, it was observed that high serotonin levels decrease heat production and/or increase heat loss and cause hypothermia[782]. Serotonin is a crucial player in hibernation and increases when the temperature drops: it is highest at the beginning of hibernation and decreases at the end of hibernation[783]. The primary mechanism through which serotonin works is probably by vasoconstriction and causing edema (build-up of fluid). Throughout the 1960s and 1970s, it was quite consistently found that more often than not, higher serotonin levels were found in people with mental retardation[784], schizophrenia[785], autism[786787], and other forms of mental abnormality and lower intelligence[788]. Most of these conditions have cold body temperatures and/or low thyroid function. One study found that 100% of severely depressed patients had decreased T3 levels[789]. These observations lead the scientist to conclude that typical anti-depressive therapy would have little effect.

It was recently found that 31 % of SIDS babies have higher serotonin levels compared to controls[790]. Serotonin has a known negative relationship with pregnancy. Elevated serotonin is often seen in toxemia[791].

Most serotonin is made in the intestines. As serotonin constricts the veins and arteries, it has the same function in the intestines. When you ingest toxins, serotonin increases to push the toxins out of your body. Serotonin is a critical player in the formation of colitis[792].

Anti-serotonin lowers context-conditioned immobility (learned helplessness) in males[793], and genetically altered mice displaying no serotonin in the brain exhibited anti-depressive effects[794]. Anti-serotonin drugs are useful in treating aspects of depression[795][796], and have the effect of being anti-fibrosis[797]. Serotonin is heavily involved in learned helplessness[798].

Serotonin is seen as a significant mediator after a stressful event, and reducing serotonin diminishes the negative aspects, such as swelling, defective blood-brain barrier, and overall pathology[799]. Probably because of the significant financial rewards from the sales of pro-serotonin medicine, its pro-inflammatory aspect in many pathologies has been neglected. Estrogen can increase serotonin[800], while vitamin A will lower it[801]. It has been noted that fish oils

(DHA) are especially useful to increase tryptophan into the brain. This is one of the reasons that omega-3 is advocated, due to its effects on the serotonin precursor tryptophan. Fish oil can increase tryptophan and serotonin in the brain[802]. Using tryptophan as a supplement has been shown to increase serotonin and consequently increase lipid peroxidation[803]. By comparison, an omega-3 deficient diet can decrease serotonin[804]. I think this is one of the reasons why tryptophan-deficient diets are considered healthy[805].

CHAPTER 13

Essential Fatty Acids Deficiency (EFAD)

"we cannot avoid the conclusion that if true fats are essential for nutrition during growth the minimum necessary must be exceedingly small"[806]

GROWTH ON DIETS POOR IN TRUE FATS. BY THOMAS B. OSBORNE AND LAFAYETTE B. MENDEL. (From the Laboratory of the Connecticut Agricultural Experiment Station and the Sheffield Laboratory of Physiological Chemistry, Yale University, New Haven.) (Received for publication, October 21, 1920).

This quote came from research conducted more than 100 years ago. The study found that adults were fine after nine months of a fat-free diet, as long as green vegetables were given [807] as they contain small amounts of ALA omega-3. At around the same time, it was found by German, American[808], and Danish scientists that rats[809], infants, youths, and adults could live with a minimum or complete exclusion of fat and that many of them thrived[810].

There is a discussion about whether the Burrs' discovery of essential fatty acids in 1929 was valid. George and Mildred Burr discovered the presence of "essential fatty acids." They found that the exclusion of these fatty acids caused rats to have, amongst other observations, dermatitis, limited growth, and, although smaller, produced a higher metabolic rate[811]. The problems associated with essential fat deficiency could be restored with as little as three drops of lard[812]. All through the last 80 plus years, scientists have argued against the accepted statement of the essentiality of these fatty acids. This author has not reached any conclusion on the subject but agrees with the statement at the beginning of the chapter that the quantities of these fats must be small. Furthermore, as observed repeatedly and described in the "eyes" segment, the body has excellent abilities to preserve long-chain unsaturated fatty acids, even in times of unsaturated fatty acid deprivation[813].

In 1929, many of the vitamins were being discovered or had not been discovered yet. In 1931, Hume found that diets could induce scaly tail in rats with and without fat and that the addition of whole dried yeast could improve mild cases of a scaly tail[814] (dried yeast contains no or micro amounts of fat, 0.001 grams). A vitamin B6 deficiency, discovered in 1934, shows the same symptoms as EFAD in rats. These include scaliness of the paws and tail, acrodynia, coarse fur, and growth retardation. Some years later, it was found that many of the ailments could be cured independently of the essential fatty acids[815], and that one of the factors was vitamin B6[816][817][818]. When EFAD and B6 deficiency were compared in monkeys, it was found that atherosclerosis was more severe in B6 deficiency than in the EFAD group[819][820]. Rats on an essential fatty acid-deficient diet show no signs of deficiency when adequate zinc is supplied[821]. Zinc deficiency shows itself as growth retardation and locomotor skills despite sufficient EFA[822], or lessen its impact[823]. Below is a summary of the supposed EFA deficiencies and a zinc deficiency:

Zinc deficiency	EFA deficiency
Growth retardation	Growth retardation
Delayed sexual maturation	Delayed sexual maturation
Infertility	Infertility
Dermal lesions	Dermal lesions
Alopecia	Alopecia
Decreased wound healing	Decreased wound healing

824

Metabolic Rate

The metabolic rate can increase as the intake of essential fatty acid decreases. The requirements for nutrients and calories increase. When rats were fed a typical diet versus fed versus EFAD rats, it was found that the EFAD rats ate about double the quantity of calories needed to sustain growth. Patients with EFAD-status can reduce their EFAD symptoms by increasing calories[825]. The omega-3 seems to be less critical than the omega-6 as in 1943; it was found that fish oil was less effective than methyl linoleate, despite its higher unsaturation[826]. When the omega-6 is excluded from the diet, the uptake of omega-3 is lessened. It seems that omega-3 is less "essential" without omega-6[827].

Problems With EFAD Research

"Undoubtedly, many if not all of the biochemical alterations in mitochondria from EFA deficient rats thus far reported are an artifact resulting from damage during isolation"[828]

1964. SMITH JA, DELUCA HF. STRUCTURAL CHANGES IN ISOLATED LIVER

MITOCHONDRIA OF RATS DURING ESSENTIAL FATTY ACID DEFICIENCY. J Cell Biol. 1964;21(1):15–26. doi:10.1083/jcb.21.1.15

It would almost be impossible to exclude some forms of omega-3 from the diets. This problem of total exclusion also exists in food research, when early on, it was found that "failure to work with a sufficiently pure diet may lead to conflicting and misleading results."[829]. The classification of EFAD as a condition made it unnecessary to be investigated or forego publishing possible positive outcomes in EFAD states (mentioned in[830]). When organisms are made deficient in PUFA, the mitochondria have ways of keeping the ratio of saturated to unsaturated fatty acids the same as in essential fatty acids[831].

"The findings support the view that altered fatty acid composition of the magnitude observed in either diabetic or essential fatty acid-deficient rats is insufficient to compromise membrane function and unlikely to provoke significant pathologic changes in capillaries within the times of observation covered by these experiments."[832]

Forrest GL, Futterman, S. Age-related changes in the retinal capillaries and the fatty acid composition of retinal tissue of normal and essential fatty acid-deficient rats. Invest Ophthalmol Vis Sci. 1972;11:760-764. In this study, only omega-6 was omitted.

EFAD Is More Anti-Inflammatory Than Fish Oil

When different animals were raised with an essential fatty acid deficiency:

- it became very difficult to produce obesity in mice even on a high-fat diet[833]

- mice had long-term protection against diet-induced liver steatosis and hypercholesterolemia[834]
- decreased anxiety in adult life in mice[835]
- lower inflammation in rats (lower than rats fed AA and DHA)[836]
- are less/not susceptible to diabetes or poisons in different animal models[837838839840]
- protects against glomerular macrophage infiltration and the ensuing proteinuria[841]
- possibly treat lupus[842]
- protects against thermal injury[843], reduces tissue damage[844]

The saturated fats seem to make mammals have more fat loss compared to essential fatty acids[845]. No essential fatty acids are needed for wound healing[846]. At the same time, it was found that omega-3 fatty acids could be detrimental to wound healing[847]. A deficiency in essential fatty acids can result in a delay in puberty (partly by lowering estrogen)[848], which is associated with many health effects. Testosterone, the hormone that declines during aging in most men, can be increased in an essential fatty acid-deficient state[849850].

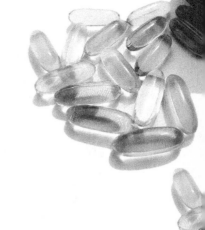

CHAPTER 14

Conclusion

As mentioned before, this book is not suggesting that the oils in fish in a regular diet are necessarily a bad thing. This book describes the possible adverse actions of these fats in concentrated form. I think that in years to come, DHA and EPA will not be derived from fish and will be generated from other sources.

The genes that generate omega-3 in algae are currently being introduced into crops to be launched in the market. Currently, the Brassica napus plants (rapeseed oil) are being experimented with. One hectare of crops can produce the equivalent of 10,000 fish in DHA quantity[851]. The genetic manipulation of plants can secure the supply for "fish oils" as current consumption levels of fish (oil) are not sustainable[852].

The science does not support the view that fish oils cannot harm. Furthermore, many researchers and scientists caution the use of these fats. As the aim of this book is to inform the reader, hopefully, you can come to your conclusion. If one decides to keep taking fish oils, at least you can understand the possible side-effects of these fragile fats.

Wishing you well in your health journey,
Youri Kruse

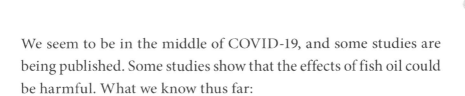

ADDENDUM

| Covid-19 & Fish Oils

We seem to be in the middle of COVID-19, and some studies are being published. Some studies show that the effects of fish oil could be harmful. What we know thus far:

A study from China shows that patients typically have low cholesterol levels and low white blood cells, neutrophils, and lymphocytes[853]. This made some scientists urge the stopping of cholesterol-lowering drugs amongst COVID-19 patients[854].

As part of the innate immune system, the natural killer (NK) together with CD8+ T cells, it is critical to control viral attacks. A study from April 2020 shows that COVID-19 patients indeed have low NK and CD8+ T cells[855].

Fish oil is known to suppress CD8 (+) T cells by reducing both its activation and proliferation[856]. In mice, fish oils lower T cells and NK cells and increase mortality rates after an influenza virus infection[857].

Scientists are now suggesting increasing or adding interferon-γ to treat COVID-19 patients[858]. Interferon-γ has a crucial role to play against coronaviruses. Animal studies show that fish oils can decrease Interferon-γ[859].

Research shows that while saturated fats are likely protective, unsaturated fat might be associated with increased mortality[860].

ENDNOTES

1   Yum, Jennie. (2007). The Effects of Breast Milk Versus Infant Formulae on Cognitive Development. JOURNAL ON DEVELOPMENTAL DISABILITIES. 13.

2   Janssen A, Baes M, Gressens P, Mannaerts GP, Declercq P, Van Veldhoven PP. Docosahexaenoic acid deficit is not a major pathogenic factor in peroxisome-deficient mice. Lab Invest. 2000;80(1):31-35. doi:10.1038/labinvest.3780005

3   Hadjiagapiou C, Spector AA. Docosahexaenoic acid metabolism and effect on prostacyclin production in endothelial cells. Arch Biochem Biophys. 1987;253(1):1-12. doi:10.1016/0003-9861(87)90631-x

4   FISHERIES RESEARCH BOARD OF CANADA Translation Series No. 2045, 'Effect of medicinal cod liver 'oil containing different amounts of aldehydes on the organism' (found here http://www.dfo-mpo.gc.ca/Library/13607.pdf). From the Fisheries and Oceans Canada

5   Tsuduki T, Honma T, Nakagawa K, Ikeda I, Miyazawa T. Long-term intake of fish oil increases oxidative stress and decreases lifespan in senescence-accelerated mice. Nutrition. 2011;27(3):334-337. doi:10.1016/j.nut.2010.05.017

6   Kang JX. Effect of ω-3 fatty acids on life span. Nutrition. 2011;27(3):333. doi:10.1016/j.nut.2010.07.011

7   Tsuduki T. Reply to Dr. Kang's letter entitled "Effect of ω-3 fatty acids on lifespan". Nutrition. 2011;27(6):731-732. doi:10.1016/j.nut.2011.03.001

8   Albert BB, Derraik JG, Cameron-Smith D, et al. Fish oil supplements in New Zealand are highly oxidised and do not meet label content of n-3 PUFA [published correction appears in Sci Rep. 2016 Nov 07;6:35092]. Sci Rep. 2015;5:7928. Published 2015 Jan 21. doi:10.1038/srep07928

9   Nichols PD, Dogan L, Sinclair A. Australian and New Zealand Fish Oil Products in 2016 Meet Label Omega-3 Claims and Are Not Oxidized. Nutrients. 2016;8(11):703. Published 2016 Nov 5. doi:10.3390/nu8110703

10 Turner R, McLean CH, Silvers KM. Are the health benefits of fish oils limited by products of oxidation?. Nutr Res Rev. 2006;19(1):53-62. doi:10.1079/NRR2006117

11 Mason RP, Sherratt SCR. Omega-3 fatty acid fish oil dietary supplements contain saturated fats and oxidized lipids that may interfere with their intended biological benefits. Biochem Biophys Res Commun. 2017;483(1):425-429. doi:10.1016/j.bbrc.2016.12.127

12 Opperman M, Benade S. Analysis of the omega-3 fatty acid content of South African fish oil supplements: a follow-up study. Cardiovasc J Afr. 2013;24(8):297-302. doi:10.5830/CVJA-2013-074

13 Opperman M, Marais de W, Spinnler Benade AJ. Analysis of omega-3 fatty acid content of South African fish oil supplements. Cardiovasc J Afr. 2011;22(6):324-329. doi:10.5830/CVJA-2010-080

14 Jackowski SA, Alvi AZ, Mirajkar A, et al. Oxidation levels of North American over-the-counter n-3 (omega-3) supplements and the influence of supplement formulation and delivery form on evaluating oxidative safety. J Nutr Sci. 2015;4:e30. Published 2015 Nov 4. doi:10.1017/jns.2015.21

15 Walter MF, Jacob RF, Bjork RE, et al. Circulating lipid hydroperoxides predict cardiovascular events in patients with stable coronary artery disease: the PREVENT study. J Am Coll Cardiol. 2008;51(12):1196-1202. doi:10.1016/j.jacc.2007.11.051

16 Tanaka, Shin-Ichiro & Miki, Tetsuo & Sha, Shoto & Hirata, Ken-Ichi & Ishikawa, Yuichi & Yokoyama, Mitsuhiro. (2011). Serum Levels of Thiobarbituric Acid-Reactive Substances are Associated with Risk of Coronary Heart Disease. Journal of atherosclerosis and thrombosis. 18. 584-91. 10.5551/jat.6585

17 Halliwell B, Chirico S. Lipid peroxidation: its mechanism, measurement, and significance. Am J Clin Nutr. 1993;57(5 Suppl):715S-725S. doi:10.1093/ajcn/57.5.715S

18 Staprāns I, Rapp JH, Pan XM, Kim KY, Feingold KR. Oxidized lipids in the diet are a source of oxidized lipid in chylomicrons of human serum. Arterioscler Thromb. 1994;14(12):1900-1905. doi:10.1161/01.atv.14.12.1900

19 Witztum JL, Steinberg D. Role of oxidized low density lipoprotein in atherogenesis. J Clin Invest. 1991;88(6):1785-1792. doi:10.1172/JCI115499

20 Iyengar NK, Mukerji B. The Quality of Medicinal Cod-Liver Oil and Its Preparations on the Indian Market. Ind Med Gaz. 1939;74(4):215-220

21 Barata C, Navarro JC, Varo I, et al. Changes in antioxidant enzyme activities, fatty acid composition and lipid peroxidation in Daphnia magna during the aging process. Comparative Biochemistry and physiology. Part B, Biochemistry & Molecular Biology. 2005 Jan;140(1):81-90. DOI: 10.1016/j.cbpc.2004.09.025

22 Ambrożewicz, Ewa & Augustyniak, Agnieszka & Gęgotek, Agnieszka & Bielawska, Katarzyna & Skrzydlewska, Elżbieta. (2013). Black-Currant Protection Against Oxidative Stress Formation. Journal of toxicology and environmental health. Part A. 76. 1293-1306. 10.1080/15287394.2013.850762

23 Palmquist, Don. (2009). Omega-3 Fatty Acids in Metabolism, Health, and Nutrition and for Modied Animal Product Foods. Professional Animal Scientist. 25. 207-249. 10.15232/S1080-7446(15)30713-0

24 D S Lin, W E Conner, Are the n-3 fatty acids from dietary fish oil deposited in the triglyceride stores of adipose tissue?, The American Journal of Clinical Nutrition, Volume 51, Issue 4, April 1990, Pages 535–539, https://doi.org/10.1093/ajcn/51.4.535

25 Lucinda KM Summers, Sophie C Barnes, Barbara A Fielding, Carine Beysen, Vera Ilic, Sandy M Humphreys, Keith N Frayn, Uptake of individual fatty acids into adipose tissue in relation to their presence in the diet; The American Journal of Clinical Nutrition, Volume 71, Issue 6, June 2000, Pages 1470–1477, https://doi.org/10.1093/ajcn/71.6.1470

26 Maruhama, Yoshisuke & Kaneko, Yoshihito & Sekine, Kohsaku & Kuroda, Tuguhisa & Mukaida, Hideaki & Ninomiya, Kazumi & Sasaki, Masataka & Takayama, Kazuo. (1992). Long-Term Storage of Fish Oil Fatty Acids in the Liver, Not Adipose Tissue, in Humans. Journal of Clinical Biochemistry and Nutrition. 12. 51-57. 10.3164/jcbn.12.51.

27 Mamalakis, G & Kafatos, A & Manios, Yannis & Kalogeropoulos, Nick & Andrikopoulos, Nikolaos. (2002). Abdominal vs buttock adipose fat: Relationships with children's serum lipids levels. European journal of clinical nutrition. 56. 1081-6. 10.1038/sj.ejcn.1601438

28 Spite M, Serhan CN. Novel lipid mediators promote resolution of acute inflammation: impact of aspirin and statins. Circ Res. 2010;107(10):1170–1184. doi:10.1161/CIRCRESAHA.110.223883

29 Jones, R., Adel-Alvarez, L., Alvarez, O.R. et al. Arachidonic acid and colorectal carcinogenesis. Mol Cell Biochem 253, 141–149 (2003). https://doi.org/10.1023/A:1026060426569

30 Wilder, R.M. (1941). Mobilize for total nutrition!. Survey Graphic, 30(7), 381. Retrieved [date accessed] from http://socialwelfare.library.vcu.edu/ eras/great-depression/mobilize-total-nutrition/

31 Products, Nutrition. (2012). Scientific Opinion on the Tolerable Upper Intake Level of eicosapentaenoic acid (EPA), docosahexaenoic acid (DHA) and docosapentaenoic acid (DPA). EFSA Journal. 10. 10.2903/j. efsa.2012.2815

32 Jenkins, G., Wainwright, L. J., Holland, R., Barrett, K. E., & Casey, J. (2014). Wrinkle reduction in post-menopausal women consuming a novel oral supplement: a double-blind placebo-controlled randomized study. International journal of cosmetic science, 36(1), 22–31. https://doi. org/10.1111/ics.12087

33 Marchioli, R., Schweiger, C., Tavazzi, L. and Valagussa, F. (2001), Efficacy of n-3 polyunsaturated fatty acids after myocardial infarction: Results of GISSI-prevenzione trial. Lipids, 36: S119-S126. doi:10.1007/ s11745-001-0694-8

34 Ghasemi Fard, Samaneh & Wang, Fenglei & Sinclair, Andrew & Elliott, Glenn & Turchini, Giovanni. (2018). How does high DHA fish oil affect health? A systematic review of evidence. Critical Reviews in Food Science and Nutrition. 59. 1-44. 10.1080/10408398.2018.1425978

35 Calder, P., Dangour, A., Diekman, C. et al. Essential fats for future health. Proceedings of the 9th Unilever Nutrition Symposium, 26–27 May 2010. Eur J Clin Nutr 64, S1–S13 (2010). https://doi.org/10.1038/ejcn.2010.242

36 Yvonne E Finnegan, Anne M Minihane, Elizabeth C Leigh-Firbank, Samantha Kew, Gert W Meijer, Reto Muggli, Philip C Calder, Christine M Williams, Plant- and marine-derived n–3 polyunsaturated fatty acids have differential effects on fasting and postprandial blood lipid concentrations and on the susceptibility of LDL to oxidative modification in moderately hyperlipidemic subjects, The American Journal of Clinical Nutrition, Volume 77, Issue 4, April 2003, Pages 783–795, https://doi.org/10.1093/ ajcn/77.4.783

37 Imhoff-Kunsch, B., Stein, A. D., Martorell, R., Parra-Cabrera, S., Romieu, I., & Ramakrishnan, U. (2011). Prenatal docosahexaenoic acid supplementation and infant morbidity: randomized controlled trial. Pediatrics, 128(3), e505–e512. https://doi.org/10.1542/peds.2010-1386

38 Mischoulon D, Nierenberg AA, Schettler PJ, et al. A double-blind, randomized controlled clinical trial comparing eicosapentaenoic acid versus

docosahexaenoic acid for depression. J Clin Psychiatry. 2015;76(1):54–61. doi:10.4088/JCP.14m08986

39   Singhal, A., Lanigan, J., Storry, C., Low, S., Birbara, T., Lucas, A., & Deanfield, J. (2013). Docosahexaenoic acid supplementation, vascular function and risk factors for cardiovascular disease: a randomized controlled trial in young adults. Journal of the American Heart Association, 2(4), e000283. https://doi.org/10.1161/JAHA.113.000283

40   Carlson SJ, Nandivada P, Chang MI, et al. The addition of medium-chain triglycerides to a purified fish oil-based diet alters inflammatory profiles in mice. Metabolism. 2015;64(2):274–282. doi:10.1016/j.metabol.2014.10.005

41   Bullon P, Battino M, Varela-Lopez A, Perez-Lopez P, Granados-Principal S, Ramirez-Tortosa MC, et al. (2013) Diets Based on Virgin Olive Oil or Fish Oil but Not on Sunflower Oil Prevent Age-Related Alveolar Bone Resorption by Mitochondrial-Related Mechanisms. PLoS ONE 8(9): e74234. https://doi.org/10.1371/journal.pone.0074234

42   Olomu JM, Baracos VE. Influence of dietary flaxseed oil on the performance, muscle protein deposition, and fatty acid composition of broiler chicks. Poult Sci. 1991;70(6):1403–1411. doi:10.3382/ps.0701403

43   Adam O, Wolfram G, Zöllner N. Effect of alpha-linolenic acid in the human diet on linoleic acid metabolism and prostaglandin biosynthesis. J Lipid Res. 1986;27(4):421–426

44   Konieczka P, Barszcz M, Choct M, Smulikowska S. The interactive effect of dietary n-6: n-3 fatty acid ratio and vitamin E level on tissue lipid peroxidation, DNA damage in intestinal epithelial cells, and gut morphology in chickens of different ages. Poult Sci. 2018;97(1):149–158. doi:10.3382/ps/pex274

45   Bonanome A, Pagnan A, Biffanti S, et al. Effect of dietary monounsaturated and polyunsaturated fatty acids on the susceptibility of plasma low density lipoproteins to oxidative modification. Arterioscler Thromb. 1992;12(4):529–533. doi:10.1161/01.atv.12.4.529

46   OBSERVATIONS ON THE BASIC NUTRITION, VITAMINS AND FOOD PREPARATIONS IN DOLPHINS. By C.F.G.W. van der Hurk, D.V.M., veterinary consultant to the Dolfinarium, Harderwijk, Bree 37, Rotterdam, Netherlands

47   http://www.nutraingredients-usa.com/Markets/ Retail-omega-3s-sales-to-hit-34.7-billion-in-2016-report-predicts

48 Blendon RJ, Benson JM, Botta MD, Weldon KJ. Users' Views of Dietary Supplements. JAMA Intern Med. 2013;173(1):74–76. doi:10.1001/2013. jamainternmed.311

49 https://nccih.nih.gov/health/omega3/introduction.htm

50 Grey A, Bolland M. Clinical Trial Evidence and Use of Fish Oil Supplements. JAMA Intern Med. 2014;174(3):460–462. doi:10.1001/jamainternmed.2013.12765

51 Saito M, Kubo K. An assessment of docosahexaenoic acid intake from the viewpoint of safety and physiological efficacy in matured rats. Ann Nutr Metab. 2002;46(5):176–181. doi:10.1159/000065404

52 Micha R, Khatibzadeh S, Shi P, et al. Global, regional, and national consumption levels of dietary fats and oils in 1990 and 2010: a systematic analysis including 266 country-specific nutrition surveys [published correction appears in BMJ. 2015;350:h1702]. BMJ. 2014;348:g2272. Published 2014 Apr 15. doi:10.1136/bmj.g2272

53 Knoll N, Kuhnt K, Kyallo FM, Kiage-Mokua BN, Jahreis G. High content of long-chain n-3 polyunsaturated fatty acids in red blood cells of Kenyan Maasai despite low dietary intake. Lipids Health Dis. 2011;10:141. Published 2011 Aug 19. doi:10.1186/1476-511X-10-141

54 Choque B, Catheline D, Delplanque B, Guesnet P, Legrand P. Dietary linoleic acid requirements in the presence of α-linolenic acid are lower than the historical 2 % of energy intake value, study in rats. Br J Nutr. 2015;113(7):1056–1068. doi:10.1017/S0007114515000094

55 Guesnet P, Lallemand SM, Alessandri JM, Jouin M, Cunnane SC. α-Linolenate reduces the dietary requirement for linoleate in the growing rat. Prostaglandins Leukot Essent Fatty Acids. 2011;85(6):353–360. doi:10.1016/j.plefa.2011.08.003

56 Bjerve KS. n-3 fatty acid deficiency in man. Journal of Internal Medicine 225 (Suppl. 1): 171–175, 1989

57 Barceló-Coblijn G, Murphy EJ, Othman R, Moghadasian MH, Kashour T, Friel JK. Flaxseed oil and fish-oil capsule consumption alters human red blood cell n-3 fatty acid composition: a multiple-dosing trial comparing 2 sources of n-3 fatty acid. Am J Clin Nutr. 2008;88(3):801–809. doi:10.1093/ajcn/88.3.801

58 Bonilla-Méndez, J. R., & Hoyos-Concha, J. L. (2018). Methods of extraction, refining and concentration of fish oil as a source of omega-3 fatty acids.

Permission from Ciencia y Tecnología Agropecuaria,19(3),645-668. https://doi.org/10.21930/rcta.vol19_num2_art:684

59   Fish meal and oil Bimbo, A.P. (2000). Fish meal and oil, in: Martin, R.E. et al. (Ed.) Marine and freshwater products handbook. pp. 541-581 In: Martin, R.E. et al. (Ed.) (2000). Marine and freshwater products handbook. Technomic Publishing Co.: Lancaster. ISBN 1-56676-889-6. XVIII, 964 pp

60   Rossi, Pablo & Grosso, N.R. & Pramparo, M.C. & Nepote, Valeria. (2012). Fractionation and concentration of omega-3 by molecular distillation. Eicosapentaenoic Acid: Sources, Health Effects and Role in Disease Prevention. 177-203

61   TY - CHAP AU - De Silva, Sena AU - Francis, David AU - Tacon, Albert PY - 2011/06/01 SP - 1 EP - 20 SN - 978-1-4398-0862-7 T1 - Fish Oils in Aquaculture; In Retrospect DO - 10.1201/9781439808634-c1 JO - Fish oil replacement and alternative lipid sources in aquaculture feeds ER –

62   EFSA Panel on Biological Hazards (BIOHAZ); Scientific Opinion on Fish Oil for Human Consumption. Food Hygiene, including Rancidity. EFSA Journal 2010;8(10):1874. [48 pp.] doi:10.2903/j.efsa.2010.1874. Available online: www.efsa.europa.eu/efsajournal.htm

63   Wijesundera, Chakra & Ceccato, Claudio & Watkins, Peter & Fagan, Peter & Fraser, Benjamin & Thienthong, Neeranat. (2012). Docosahexaenoic Acid is More Stable to Oxidation when Located at the sn-2 Position of Triacylglycerol Compared to sn-1(3). Journal of the American Oil Chemists Society. 85. 543-548. 10.1007/s11746-008-1224-z

64   Ritter, Jenna & Budge, Suzanne & Jovica, Fabiola & Reid, Anna-Jean. (2015). Oxidation Rates of Triacylglycerol and Ethyl Ester Fish Oils. Journal of the American Oil Chemists' Society. 92. 10.1007/s11746-015-2612-9

65   Thies F, Garry JM, Yaqoob P, et al. Association of n-3 polyunsaturated fatty acids with stability of atherosclerotic plaques: a randomised controlled trial. Lancet. 2003;361(9356):477–485. doi:10.1016/S0140-6736(03)12468-3

66   Vilaseca J, Salas A, Guarner F, Rodríguez R, Martínez M, Malagelada JR. Dietary fish oil reduces progression of chronic inflammatory lesions in a rat model of granulomatous colitis. Gut. 1990;31(5):539–544. doi:10.1136/gut.31.5.539

67   Noreen EE, Sass MJ, Crowe ML, Pabon VA, Brandauer J, Averill LK. Effects of supplemental fish oil on resting metabolic rate, body composition, and salivary cortisol in healthy adults. J Int Soc Sports Nutr. 2010;7:31. Published 2010 Oct 8. doi:10.1186/1550-2783-7-31

68 Maia, M.R., Chaudhary, L.C., Bestwick, C.S. et al. Toxicity of unsaturated fatty acids to the biohydrogenating ruminal bacterium, Butyrivibrio fibrisolvens. BMC Microbiol 10, 52 (2010). https://doi.org/10.1186/1471-2180-10-52

69 Andrews JS, Griffith WH, Mead JF, Stein RA. Toxicity of air-oxidized soybean oil. J Nutr. 1960;70:199–210. doi:10.1093/jn/70.2.199

70 Fish lipids in animal nutrition. Author: Johannes Opstvedt; International Fishmeal and Oil Manufacturers Association. Publisher: St. Albans, Hertfordshire : International Fishmeal & Oil Manufacturers Association, 1985. Series: IFOMA technical bulletin, no. 22

71 Domínguez Z, Bosch V. Dietary fish oil affects food intake, growth and hematologic values of weanling rats. Arch Latinoam Nutr. 1994;44(2):92–97

72 Verschuren PM, Houtsmuller UM, Zevenbergen JL. Evaluation of vitamin E requirement and food palatability in rabbits fed a purified diet with a high fish oil content. Lab Anim. 1990;24(2):164–171. doi:10.1258/002367790780890167

73 Verschuren PM, Houtsmuller UM, Zevenbergen JL. Evaluation of vitamin E requirement and food palatability in rabbits fed a purified diet with a high fish oil content. Lab Anim. 1990;24(2):164–171. doi:10.1258/002367790780890167

74 Weindruch R, Walford RL, Fligiel S, Guthrie D. The retardation of aging in mice by dietary restriction: longevity, cancer, immunity and lifetime energy intake. J Nutr. 1986;116(4):641–654. doi:10.1093/jn/116.4.641

75 F. C. JAGER, LINOLEIC ACID INTAKE AND VITAMIN E REQUIREMENT. Thesis Unilever Research - Vlaardingen -1973

76 Fritsche KL, Johnston PV. Rapid autoxidation of fish oil in diets without added antioxidants. J Nutr. 1988;118(4):425–426. doi:10.1093/jn/118.4.425

77 Dodge JT, Phillips GB. Autoxidation as a cause of altered lipid distribution in extracts from human red cells. J Lipid Res. 1966;7(3):387–395

78 BERNHEIM F, BERNHEIM ML, WILBUR KM. The reaction between thiobarbituric acid and the oxidation products of certain lipides. J Biol Chem. 1948;174(1):257–264

79 1978. Fisk. Dir. Skr.; Srr. Ernaring I: No. 4, 105-1 16. FATTY ACID COMPOSITIONS OF FISH FATS. COMPARISONS BASED ON EIGHT FATTY ACIDS. BY GEORG LAMBERTSEN Directorate of Fisheries, Bergen, Norway.

80 Varela-Lopez A, Pérez-López MP, Ramirez-Tortosa CL, et al. Gene pathways associated with mitochondrial function, oxidative stress and telomere length are differentially expressed in the liver of rats fed lifelong on virgin olive, sunflower or fish oils. J Nutr Biochem. 2018;52:36–44. doi:10.1016/j.jnutbio.2017.09.007

81 Patel BP, Safdar A, Raha S, Tarnopolsky MA, Hamadeh MJ (2010) Caloric Restriction Shortens Lifespan through an Increase in Lipid Peroxidation, Inflammation and Apoptosis in the G93A Mouse, an Animal Model of ALS. PLoS ONE 5(2): e9386. https://doi.org/10.1371/journal.pone.0009386

82 Alizadeh A, Taleb Z, Ebrahimi B, et al. Dietary Vitamin E Is More Effective than Omega-3 and Omega-6 Fatty Acid for Improving The Kinematic Characteristics of Rat Sperm. Cell J. 2016;18(2):262–270. doi:10.22074/cellj.2016.4322

83 Mezzetti A, Zuliani G, Romano F, et al. Vitamin E and lipid peroxide plasma levels predict the risk of cardiovascular events in a group of healthy very old people. J Am Geriatr Soc. 2001;49(5):533–537. doi:10.1046/j.1532-5415.2001.49110.x

84 Patel BP, Safdar A, Raha S, Tarnopolsky MA, Hamadeh MJ (2010) Caloric Restriction Shortens Lifespan through an Increase in Lipid Peroxidation, Inflammation and Apoptosis in the G93A Mouse, an Animal Model of ALS. PLoS ONE 5(2): e9386. https://doi.org/10.1371/journal.pone.0009386

85 Harris PL, Embree ND. QUANTITATIVE CONSIDERATION OF THE EFFECT OF POLYUNSATURATED FATTY ACID CONTENT OF THE DIET UPON THE REQUIREMENTS FOR VITAMIN E. Am J Clin Nutr. 1963;13(6):385–392. doi:10.1093/ajcn/13.6.385

86 Muggli R. Physiological requirements of vitamin E as a function of the amount and type of polyunsaturated fatty acid. World Rev Nutr Diet. 1994;75:166–168. doi:10.1159/000423574

87 Villaverde C, Baucells MD, Manzanilla EG, Barroeta AC. High levels of dietary unsaturated fat decrease alpha-tocopherol content of whole body, liver, and plasma of chickens without variations in intestinal apparent absorption. Poult Sci. 2008;87(3):497–505

88 Bässler KH. On the problematic nature of vitamin E requirements: net vitamin E. Z Ernahrungswiss. 1991;30(3):174–180. doi:10.1007/bf01610340

89 Maras JE, Bermudez OI, Qiao N, Bakun PJ, Boody-Alter EL, Tucker KL. Intake of alpha-tocopherol is limited among US adults. J Am Diet Assoc. 2004;104(4):567–575. doi:10.1016/j.jada.2004.01.004

90 Panemangalore M, Lee CJ. Evaluation of the indices of retinol and alpha-tocopherol status in free-living elderly. J Gerontol. 1992;47(3):B98–B104. doi:10.1093/geronj/47.3.b98

91 Hiki M, Miyazaki T, Shimada K, et al. Significance of Serum Polyunsaturated Fatty Acid Level Imbalance in Patients with Acute Venous Thromboembolism. J Atheroscler Thromb. 2017;24(10):1016–1022. doi:10.5551/jat.37424

92 Wang YE, Tseng VL, Yu F, Caprioli J, Coleman AL. Association of Dietary Fatty Acid Intake With Glaucoma in the United States. JAMA Ophthalmol. 2018;136(2):141–147. doi:10.1001/jamaophthalmol.2017.5702

93 Rabini RA, Moretti N, Staffolani R, et al. Reduced susceptibility to peroxidation of erythrocyte plasma membranes from centenarians. Exp Gerontol. 2002;37(5):657–663. doi:10.1016/s0531-5565(02)00006-2

94 Wander RC, Hall JA, Gradin JL, Du SH, Jewell DE. The ratio of dietary (n-6) to (n-3) fatty acids influences immune system function, eicosanoid metabolism, lipid peroxidation and vitamin E status in aged dogs. J Nutr. 1997;127(6):1198–1205. doi:10.1093/jn/127.6.1198

95 Shefer-Weinberg, Diana & Sasson, Shlomo & Schwartz, Betty & Argov-Argaman, Nurit & Tirosh, Oren. (2017). Deleterious effect of n-3 polyunsaturated fatty acids in non-alcoholic steatohepatitis in the fat-1 mouse model. Clinical Nutrition Experimental. 12. 10.1016/j.yclnex.2016.12.003

96 Konieczka P, Barszcz M, Choct M, Smulikowska S. The interactive effect of dietary n-6: n-3 fatty acid ratio and vitamin E level on tissue lipid peroxidation, DNA damage in intestinal epithelial cells, and gut morphology in chickens of different ages. Poult Sci. 2018;97(1):149–158. doi:10.3382/ps/pex274

97 Castro-Correia, C. & Sousa, S. & Norberto, Sónia & Matos, C. & Domingues, Valentina & Fontoura, M. & Calhau, Conceição. (2017). The Fatty Acid Profile in Patients with Newly Diagnosed Diabetes: Why It Could Be Unsuspected. International Journal of Pediatrics. 2017. 1-5. 10.1155/2017/6424186.

98 Watanabe S, Tsuneyama K. Eicosapentaenoic acid attenuates hepatic accumulation of cholesterol esters but aggravates liver injury and inflammation in mice fed a cholate-supplemented high-fat diet. J Toxicol Sci. 2013;38(3):379–390. doi:10.2131/jts.38.379

99 Muhlhausler BS, Miljkovic D, Fong L, Xian CJ, Duthoit E, Gibson RA. Maternal omega-3 supplementation increases fat mass in male and female rat offspring. Front Genet. 2011;2:48. Published 2011 Jul 21. doi:10.3389/fgene.2011.00048

100 Grúz, Petr & Shimizu, Masatomi & Sugiyama, Kei-Ichi & Honma, Masamitsu. (2017). Mutagenicity of ω-3 fatty acid peroxidation products in the Ames test. Mutation Research/Genetic Toxicology and Environmental Mutagenesis. 819. 10.1016/j.mrgentox.2017.05.004

101 Lee JS, Cole SR, Achenbach CJ, Dittmer DP, Richardson DB, Miller WC, et al. (2018) Cancer risk in HIV patients with incomplete viral suppression after initiation of antiretroviral therapy. PLoS ONE 13(6): e0197665. https://doi.org/10.1371/journal.pone.0197665

102 Adami J, Gäbel H, Lindelöf B, et al. Cancer risk following organ transplantation: a nationwide cohort study in Sweden. Br J Cancer. 2003;89(7):1221–1227. doi:10.1038/sj.bjc.6601219

103 Petersen DR, Saba LM, Sayin VI, Papagiannakopoulos T, Schmidt EE, Merrill GF, et al. (2018) Elevated Nrf-2 responses are insufficient to mitigate protein carbonylation in hepatospecific PTEN deletion mice. PLoS ONE 13(5): e0198139. https://doi.org/10.1371/journal.pone.0198139

104 Kris-Etherton PM, Taylor DS, Yu-Poth S, et al. Polyunsaturated fatty acids in the food chain in the United States. Am J Clin Nutr. 2000;71(1 Suppl):179S–88S. doi:10.1093/ajcn/71.1.179S

105 Letter to the Editor Gibson, Robert et al. Prostaglandins, Leukotrienes and Essential Fatty Acids, Volume 85, Issue 6, 403 – 404

106 Rylander C, Sandanger TM, Engeset D, Lund E. Consumption of lean fish reduces the risk of type 2 diabetes mellitus: a prospective population based cohort study of Norwegian women. PLoS One. 2014;9(2):e89845. Published 2014 Feb 24. doi:10.1371/journal.pone.0089845

107 Morris MC, Evans DA, Tangney CC, Bienias JL, Wilson RS. Fish consumption and cognitive decline with age in a large community study. Arch Neurol. 2005;62(12):1849–1853. doi:10.1001/archneur.62.12.noc50161

108 Owen AJ, Magliano DJ, O'Dea K, Barr EL, Shaw JE. Polyunsaturated fatty acid intake and risk of cardiovascular mortality in a low fish-consuming population: a prospective cohort analysis. Eur J Nutr. 2016;55(4):1605–1613. doi:10.1007/s00394-015-0979-x

109 Werner, T., Kumar, R., Horvath, I., Scheers, N., & Wittung-Stafshede, P. (2018). Abundant fish protein inhibits α-synuclein amyloid formation. Scientific reports, 8(1), 5465. (2018). doi:10.1038/s41598-018-23850-0

110 Visioli, F., Risé, P., Barassi, M.C. et al. Dietary intake of fish vs. formulations leads to higher plasma concentrations of n–3 fatty acids. Lipids 38, 415–418 (2003). https://doi.org/10.1007/s11745-003-1077-x

111 Helland IB, Smith L, Saarem K, Saugstad OD, Drevon CA. Maternal supplementation with very-long-chain n-3 fatty acids during pregnancy and lactation augments children's IQ at 4 years of age. Pediatrics. 2003;111(1):e39–e44. doi:10.1542/peds.111.1.e39

112 Helland, Ingrid B. et al. "Effect of supplementing pregnant and lactating mothers with n-3 very-long-chain fatty acids on children's IQ and body mass index at 7 years of age." Pediatrics 122 2 (2008): e472-9

113 D.N.S Kerr, Hypercalcemia and metastatic calcification, Cardiovascular Research, Volume 36, Issue 3, December 1997, Pages 293–297, https://doi.org/10.1016/S0008-6363(97)00243-5

114 RICKETS 1925. Rickets*. By DR. JOSEPH GARLAND, Boston, Mass. Visiting Physician to Children's Medical Department, Massachusetts General Hospital; Assistant in Pediatrics, Harvard Medical School. March 26, 1925 Boston Med Surg J 1925; 192:581-588 DOI: 10.1056/NEJM192503261921301

115 Holmes, A. D. Studies of the Vitamin Potency of Cod Liver Oils. II. The effect of season on the vitamin e potency of cod liver oils. Spring Oil. Presented at Fall Meeting (1922) American Chemical Society

116 Ind. Eng. Chem. 1924, 16, 3, 295-297 Publication Date:March 1, 1924 https://doi.org/10.1021/ie50171a030

117 Norris, Earl R. and Anna E. Church. "THE TOXIC EFFECT OF FISH LIVER OILS, AND THE ACTION OF VITAMIN B."1930 (2003).

118 AGDUHR, E. (1926), Changes in the Organism caused by Cod-liver Oil added to the Food.. Acta Pædiatrica, 6: 165-179. doi:10.1111/j.1651-2227.1926.tb09343.x

119 Agduhr, E. The changes in the heart through the presence of cod liver oil in the food. Actappaediatrica 5, 319, 1926

120 THE TOXIC EFFECT OF FISH LIVER OILS, AND THE ACTION OF VITAMIN B. BY EARL R. NORRIS AND ANNA E. CHURCH. (From the Division of Biochemistry, University of Washington, Seattle.) (Received for publication, August 6, 1930.)

121 Simons, E. J., L. O. Buxton, and H. B. Coleman, 1940. Relation of Peroxide Formation to Destruction of Vitamin A in Fish Liver Oils. Ind. Eng. Chem. 23., 706-708

122 INACTIVATION OF BIOTIN BY RANCID FATS* BY P. L. PAVCEK AND G. M. SHULL (From the Department of Biochemistry, College of Agriculture, University of Wisconsin, Madison) (Received for publication, September 5, 1942)

123 Role of unsaturated fatty acids in changes of adipose and dental tissues in vitamin E deficiency.Author(s) : DAM, H.; GRANADOS, H. Author Affiliation : Sch. Med. Dent., Univ. Rochester, N.Y. Journal article : Science (Washington) 1945 Vol.102 pp.327-328

124 Piché LA, Draper HH, Cole PD. Malondialdehyde excretion by subjects consuming cod liver oil vs a concentrate of n-3 fatty acids. Lipids. 1988;23(4):370–371. doi:10.1007/bf02537352l

125 Wójcik OP, Koenig KL, Zeleniuch-Jacquotte A, Costa M, Chen Y. The potential protective effects of taurine on coronary heart disease. Atherosclerosis. 2010;208(1):19–25. doi:10.1016/j.atherosclerosis.2009.06.002

126 Ripps H, Shen W. Review: taurine: a "very essential" amino acid. Mol Vis. 2012;18:2673–2686

127 127 Ahmadian M, Roshan VD, Aslani E, Stannard SR. Taurine supplementation has anti-atherogenic and anti-inflammatory effects before and after incremental exercise in heart failure. Ther Adv Cardiovasc Dis. 2017;11(7):185–194. doi:10.1177/1753944717711138

128 Matsushima Y, Sekine T, Kondo Y, et al. Effects of taurine on serum cholesterol levels and development of atherosclerosis in spontaneously hyperlipidaemic mice. Clin Exp Pharmacol Physiol. 2003;30(4):295–299. doi:10.1046/j.1440-1681.2003.03828.x

129 El Idrissi A, Okeke E, Yan X, Sidime F, Neuwirth LS. Taurine regulation of blood pressure and vasoactivity. Adv Exp Med Biol. 2013;775:407–425. doi:10.1007/978-1-4614-6130-2_31

130 Park T, Lee K. Dietary taurine supplementation reduces plasma and liver cholesterol and triglyceride levels in rats fed a high-cholesterol or a cholesterol-free diet. Adv Exp Med Biol. 1998;442:319–325. doi:10.1007/978-1-4899-0117-0_40

131 Yokogoshi H, Mochizuki H, Nanami K, Hida Y, Miyachi F, Oda H. Dietary taurine enhances cholesterol degradation and reduces serum and liver

cholesterol concentrations in rats fed a high-cholesterol diet. J Nutr. 1999;129(9):1705–1712. doi:10.1093/jn/129.9.1705

132 Pasantes, Herminia & Quesada, Octavio & Alcocer, L. & Olea, R.. (1989). Taurine content in foods. Nutrition Reports International. 40. 793-801

133 Masuda M, Horisaka K, Koeda T. [Role of taurine in neutrophil function]. Nihon Yakurigaku zasshi. Folia Pharmacologica Japonica. 1984 Sep;84(3):283-292

134 Wu JY, Prentice H. Role of taurine in the central nervous system. J Biomed Sci. 2010;17 Suppl 1(Suppl 1):S1. Published 2010 Aug 24. doi:10.1186/1423-0127-17-S1-S1

135 Akil M, Bicer M, Menevse E, Baltaci AK, Mogulkoc R. Selenium supplementation prevents lipid peroxidation caused by arduous exercise in rat brain tissue. Bratisl Lek Listy. 2011;112(6):314–317

136 Baker, Robert & Baker, Susan & LaRosa, K & Whitney, C & Newburger, Peter. (1993). Selenium Regulation of Glutathione Peroxidase in Human Hepatoma Cell Line Hep3B. Archives of biochemistry and biophysics. 304. 53-7. 10.1006/abbi.1993.1320

137 Younes M, Siegers CP. Mechanistic aspects of enhanced lipid peroxidation following glutathione depletion in vivo. Chem Biol Interact. 1981;34(3):257–266. doi:10.1016/0009-2797(81)90098-3

138 Bellisola G, Galassini S, Moschini G, Poli G, Perona G, Guidi G. Selenium and glutathione peroxidase variations induced by polyunsaturated fatty acids oral supplementation in humans. Clin Chim Acta. 1992;205(1-2):75–85. doi:10.1016/s0009-8981(05)80002-6

139 Rita Cardoso B, Silva Bandeira V, Jacob-Filho W, Franciscato Cozzolino SM. Selenium status in elderly: relation to cognitive decline. J Trace Elem Med Biol. 2014;28(4):422–426. doi:10.1016/j.jtemb.2014.08.009

140 Wakimoto, Toshiyuki & Kondo, Hikaru & Nii, Hirohiko & Kimura, Kaori & Egami, Yoko & Oka, Yusuke & Yoshida, Masae & Kida, Eri & Ye, Yiping & Akahoshi, Saeko & Asakawa, Tomohiro & Matsumura, Koichi & Ishida, Hitoshi & Nukaya, Haruo & Tsuji, Kuniro & Kan, Toshiyuki & Abe, Ikuro. (2011). Furan fatty acid as an anti-inflammatory component from the green-lipped mussel Perna canaliculus. Proceedings of the National Academy of Sciences of the United States of America. 108. 17533-7. 10.1073/pnas.1110577108

141 Wahl, H.G., Liebich, H.M. and Hoffmann, A. (1994), Identification of fatty acid methyl esters as minor components of fish oil by multidimensional

GC-MSD: New furan fatty acids. J. High Resol. Chromatogr., 17: 308-311. doi:10.1002/jhrc.1240170505

142 Erkkilä AT, Schwab US, de Mello VD, et al. Effects of fatty and lean fish intake on blood pressure in subjects with coronary heart disease using multiple medications. Eur J Nutr. 2008;47(6):319–328. doi:10.1007/s00394-008-0728-5

143 Tørris C, Molin M, Cvancarova MS. Lean fish consumption is associated with lower risk of metabolic syndrome: a Norwegian cross sectional study. BMC Public Health. 2016;16:347. Published 2016 Apr 19. doi:10.1186/s12889-016-3014-0

144 Brantsæter AL, Englund-Ögge L, Haugen M, et al. Maternal intake of seafood and supplementary long chain n-3 poly-unsaturated fatty acids and preterm delivery [published correction appears in BMC Pregnancy Childbirth. 2017 Feb 10;17 (1):61]. BMC Pregnancy Childbirth. 2017;17(1):41. Published 2017 Jan 19. doi:10.1186/s12884-017-1225-8

145 Tørris C, Molin M, Småstuen MC. Lean Fish Consumption Is Associated with Beneficial Changes in the Metabolic Syndrome Components: A 13-Year Follow-Up Study from the Norwegian Tromsø Study. Nutrients. 2017;9(3):247. Published 2017 Mar 8. doi:10.3390/nu9030247

146 Norwegian Food Safety Authority, Norwegian Directorate of Health and the University of Oslo, Food composition table 2006 www.matportalen.no/matvaretabellen

147 Telle-Hansen VH, Larsen LN, Høstmark AT, et al. Daily intake of cod or salmon for 2 weeks decreases the 18:1n-9/18:0 ratio and serum triacylglycerols in healthy subjects [published correction appears in Lipids. 2012 Jul;47(7):755-6]. Lipids. 2012;47(2):151–160. doi:10.1007/s11745-011-3637-y

148 Calculated from : Møller, A., Saxholt, E., Christensen, A.T., Hartkopp, H.B., Hess Ygil, K.: Danish Food Composition Databank, revision 6.0, Food Informatics, Depa rtment of Nutrition, Danish Institute for Food and Veterinary Research, June 2005 - http://www.foodcomp.dk

149 Phleger, Charles F.. "Buoyancy in Marine Fishes: Direct and Indirect Role of Lipids'." (1998)

150 Nurk E, Drevon CA, Refsum H, et al. Cognitive performance among the elderly and dietary fish intake: the Hordaland Health Study. Am J Clin Nutr. 2007;86(5):1470–1478. doi:10.1093/ajcn/86.5.1470

151 Craig L. Frank et al. The relationship between lipid peroxidation, hibernation, and food selection in mammals. Integrative & Comparative Biology (1998) 38 (2): 341-349. By permission of Oxford University Press on behalf of Society for Integrative and Comparative Biology. Available at: https://academic.oup.com/icb/article/38/2/341/213970?searchresult=1

152 Farkas T, Kitajka K, Fodor E, et al. Docosahexaenoic acid-containing phospholipid molecular species in brains of vertebrates. Proc Natl Acad Sci U S A. 2000;97(12):6362–6366. doi:10.1073/pnas.120157297

153 Contreras C, Franco M, Place NJ, Nespolo RF. The effects of poly-unsaturated fatty acids on the physiology of hibernation in a South American marsupial, Dromiciops gliroides. Comp Biochem Physiol A Mol Integr Physiol. 2014;177:62–69. doi:10.1016/j.cbpa.2014.07.004

154 Giudetti AM, Sabetta S, di Summa R, et al. Differential effects of coconut oil- and fish oil-enriched diets on tricarboxylate carrier in rat liver mitochondria. J Lipid Res. 2003;44(11):2135–2141. doi:10.1194/jlr.M300237-JLR200

155 Kjaer MA, Todorcević M, Torstensen BE, Vegusdal A, Ruyter B. Dietary n-3 HUFA affects mitochondrial fatty acid beta-oxidation capacity and susceptibility to oxidative stress in Atlantic salmon. Lipids. 2008;43(9):813–827. doi:10.1007/s11745-008-3208-z

156 Safiulina D, Veksler V, Zharkovsky A, Kaasik A. Loss of mitochondrial membrane potential is associated with increase in mitochondrial volume: physiological role in neurones. J Cell Physiol. 2006;206(2):347–353. doi:10.1002/jcp.20476

157 Gerson AR, Brown JC, Thomas R, Bernards MA, Staples JF. Effects of dietary polyunsaturated fatty acids on mitochondrial metabolism in mammalian hibernation. J Exp Biol. 2008;211(Pt 16):2689–2699. doi:10.1242/jeb.013714

158 Surett, M.E. & CROSET, M & Lokesh, Belur & Kinsella, J.E.. (1990). The fatty acid composition and Na+-K-K+ atpase activity of kidney microsomes from mice consuming diets of varying docosahexaenoic acid and linoleic acid ratios. Nutrition Research - NUTR RES. 10. 211-218. 10.1016/S0271-5317(05)80608-6

159 Mayol V, Duran MJ, Gerbi A, et al. Cholesterol and omega-3 fatty acids inhibit Na, K-ATPase activity in human endothelial cells. Atherosclerosis. 1999;142(2):327–333. doi:10.1016/s0021-9150(98)00253-6

160 Thomas CE, Reed DJ. Radical-induced inactivation of kidney Na+,K(+)-ATPase: sensitivity to membrane lipid peroxidation and the protective

effect of vitamin E. Arch Biochem Biophys. 1990;281(1):96–105. doi:10.1016/0003-9861(90)90418-x

161 Yamaoka S, Urade R, Kito M. Mitochondrial function in rats is affected by modification of membrane phospholipids with dietary sardine oil. J Nutr. 1988;118(3):290–296. doi:10.1093/jn/118.3.290

162 Sullivan EM, Pennington ER, Sparagna GC, et al. Docosahexaenoic acid lowers cardiac mitochondrial enzyme activity by replacing linoleic acid in the phospholipidome. J Biol Chem. 2018;293(2):466–483. doi:10.1074/jbc. M117.812834

163 Figueroa-García MdC, Espinosa-García MT, Martinez-Montes F, Palomar-Morales M, Mejía-Zepeda R (2015) Even a Chronic Mild Hyperglycemia Affects Membrane Fluidity and Lipoperoxidation in Placental Mitochondria in Wistar Rats. PLoS ONE 10(12): e0143778. https://doi.org/10.1371/journal. pone.0143778

164 Müller HL, Kirchgessner M. Thermogenese und Energieverwertung bei Verabreichung von Olivenöl und Fischöl im Modellversuch an Sauen [Thermogenesis and energy utilization of olive oil and fish oil in a model study with sows]. Z Ernahrungswiss. 1995;34(2):143–150. doi:10.1007/ bf01636948

165 Kirchgessner M, Müller HL. Thermogenese im Bereich der Uberernährung bei Verabreichung von Olivenöl und Fischöl im Modellversuch an Sauen [Thermogenesis in overfeeding with administration of olive oil and fish oil in a swine model study]. Z Ernahrungswiss. 1995;34(3):206–213. doi:10.1007/bf01623159

166 Mohan PF, Phillips FC, Cleary MP. Metabolic effects of coconut, safflower, or menhaden oil feeding in lean and obese Zucker rats. Br J Nutr. 1991;66(2):285–299. doi:10.1079/bjn19910032

167 Kargar S, Ghorbani GR, Fievez V, Schingoethe DJ. Performance, bioenergetic status, and indicators of oxidative stress of environmentally heat-loaded Holstein cows in response to diets inducing milk fat depression. J Dairy Sci. 2015;98(7):4772–4784. doi:10.3168/jds.2014-9100

168 Yamaoka S, Urade R, Kito M. Mitochondrial function in rats is affected by modification of membrane phospholipids with dietary sardine oil. J Nutr. 1988;118(3):290–296. doi:10.1093/jn/118.3.290

169 Giudetti AM, Sabetta S, di Summa R, et al. Differential effects of coconut oil- and fish oil-enriched diets on tricarboxylate carrier in rat

liver mitochondria. J Lipid Res. 2003;44(11):2135–2141. doi:10.1194/jlr. M300237-JLR200

170 Siculella L, Sabetta S, Giudetti AM, Gnoni GV. Hypothyroidism reduces tricarboxylate carrier activity and expression in rat liver mitochondria by reducing nuclear transcription rate and splicing efficiency. J Biol Chem. 2006;281(28):19072–19080. doi:10.1074/jbc.M507237200

171 Zara V, Gnoni GV. Effect of starvation on the activity of the mitochondrial tricarboxylate carrier. Biochim Biophys Acta. 1995;1239(1):33–38. doi:10.1016/0005-2736(95)00125-m

172 Peoples, Gregory & Mclennan, Peter & Howe, Peter & Groeller, Herbert. (2008). Fish Oil Reduces Heart Rate and Oxygen Consumption During Exercise. Journal of cardiovascular pharmacology. 52. 540-7. 10.1097/FJC.0b013e3181911913

173 Kang JX. Reduction of heart rate by omega-3 fatty acids and the potential underlying mechanisms. Front Physiol. 2012;3:416. Published 2012 Oct 30. doi:10.3389/fphys.2012.00416

174 Berger MM, Tappy L, Revelly JP, et al. Fish oil after abdominal aorta aneurysm surgery [published correction appears in Eur J Clin Nutr. 2009 Feb;63(2):302]. Eur J Clin Nutr. 2008;62(9):1116–1122. doi:10.1038/sj.ejcn.1602817

175 Sullivan EM, Pennington ER, Sparagna GC, et al. Docosahexaenoic acid lowers cardiac mitochondrial enzyme activity by replacing linoleic acid in the phospholipidome. J Biol Chem. 2018;293(2):466–483. doi:10.1074/jbc. M117.812834

176 Kjaer MA, Todorcević M, Torstensen BE, Vegusdal A, Ruyter B. Dietary n-3 HUFA affects mitochondrial fatty acid beta-oxidation capacity and susceptibility to oxidative stress in Atlantic salmon. Lipids. 2008;43(9):813–827. doi:10.1007/s11745-008-3208-z

177 Panov, Alexander. (2017). Mitochondrial Production of Perhydroxyl Radical (HO2•) as Inducer of Aging and Age-Related Pathologies. Journal of Biochemistry and Biophysics. 1. 10.15744/2576-7623.1.105

178 Lesnefsky EJ, Hoppel CL. Cardiolipin as an oxidative target in cardiac mitochondria in the aged rat. Biochim Biophys Acta. 2008;1777(7-8):1020–1027. doi:10.1016/j.bbabio.2008.05.444

179 Sullivan EM, Pennington ER, Sparagna GC, et al. Docosahexaenoic acid lowers cardiac mitochondrial enzyme activity by replacing linoleic acid in

the phospholipidome. J Biol Chem. 2018;293(2):466–483. doi:10.1074/jbc. M117.812834

180 Kagan VE, Bayir A, Bayir H, et al. Mitochondria-targeted disruptors and inhibitors of cytochrome c/cardiolipin peroxidase complexes: a new strategy in anti-apoptotic drug discovery. Mol Nutr Food Res. 2009;53(1):104–114. doi:10.1002/mnfr.200700402

181 Petrosillo G, Ruggiero FM, Paradies G. Role of reactive oxygen species and cardiolipin in the release of cytochrome c from mitochondria. FASEB J. 2003;17(15):2202–2208. doi:10.1096/fj.03-0012com

182 Paradies G, Petrosillo G, Ruggiero FM. Cardiolipin-dependent decrease of cytochrome c oxidase activity in heart mitochondria from hypothyroid rats. Biochim Biophys Acta. 1997;1319(1):5–8. doi:10.1016/ s0005-2728(97)00012-1

183 Schlame M, Hostetler KY. Cardiolipin synthase from mammalian mitochondria. Biochim Biophys Acta. 1997;1348(1-2):207–213. doi:10.1016/ s0005-2760(97)00119-7

184 Mohan PF, Phillips FC, Cleary MP. Metabolic effects of coconut, safflower, or menhaden oil feeding in lean and obese Zucker rats. Br J Nutr. 1991;66(2):285–299. doi:10.1079/bjn199100

185 Lim CF, Munro SL, Wynne KN, Topliss DJ, Stockigt JR. Influence of nonesterified fatty acids and lysolecithins on thyroxine binding to thyroxine-binding globulin and transthyretin. Thyroid. 1995;5(4):319–324. doi:10.1089/thy.1995.5.319

186 Tabachnick M, Korcek L. Effect of long-chain fatty acids on the binding of thyroxine and triiodothyronine to human thyroxine-binding globulin. Biochim Biophys Acta. 1986;881(2):292–296. doi:10.1016/0304-4165(86)90016-4

187 Greenbaum AL, Walters E, McLean P. The effect of thyroidectomy on the pattern of fatty acids synthesized by mammary gland from lactating rats. Biochem J. 1967;103(3):720–723. doi:10.1042/bj1030720

188 Benvenga S, Li Calzi L, Robbins J. Effect of free fatty acids and nonlipid inhibitors of thyroid hormone binding in the immunoradiometric assay of thyroxin-binding globulin. Clin Chem. 1987;33(10):1752–1755

189 Clarke SD, Hembree J. Inhibition of triiodothyronine's induction of rat liver lipogenic enzymes by dietary fat. J Nutr. 1990;120(6):625–630. doi:10.1093/ jn/120.6.625

190 Scheele, Cor W. Ascites in chickens : oxygen consumption and requirement related to its occurrence / Cor W. Scheele - [S.I. : s.n.] Thesis Landbouwuniversiteit Wageningen. - With réf. - With summary in Dutch. ISBN 90-5485-499-5

191 Taraghijou P, Safaeiyan A, Mobasseri M, Ostadrahimi A. The effect of n-3 long chain fatty acids supplementation on plasma peroxisome proliferator activated receptor gamma and thyroid hormones in obesity. J Res Med Sci. 2012;17(10):942–946

192 Ramandeep K, Kapil G, Harkiran K. Correlation of enhanced oxidative stress with altered thyroid profile: Probable role in spontaneous abortion. Int J Appl Basic Med Res. 2017;7(1):20–25. doi:10.4103/2229-516X.198514

193 Azizi F, Mannix JE, Howard D, Nelson RA. Effect of winter sleep on pituitary-thyroid axis in American black bear. The American Journal of Physiology. 1979 Sep;237(3):E227-30. DOI: 10.1152/ajpendo.1979.237.3.e227

194 Kim TH, Kim KW, Ahn HY, et al. Effect of seasonal changes on the transition between subclinical hypothyroid and euthyroid status. J Clin Endocrinol Metab. 2013;98(8):3420–3429. doi:10.1210/jc.2013-1607

195 Leppäluoto J, Sikkilä K, Hassi J. Seasonal variation of serum TSH and thyroid hormones in males living in subarctic environmental conditions. Int J Circumpolar Health. 1998;57 Suppl 1:383–385

196 Jiang, Yue & Chen, Feng. (2012). Effects of temperature and temperature shift on docosahexaenoic acid production by the marine microalge Crypthecodinium cohnii. Journal of the American Oil Chemists' Society. 77. 613-617. 10.1007/s11746-000-0099-0

197 Aguilar PS, de Mendoza D. Control of fatty acid desaturation: a mechanism conserved from bacteria to humans. Mol Microbiol. 2006;62(6):1507–1514. doi:10.1111/j.1365-2958.2006.05484.x

198 28th Lipidforum Symposium, Reykjavik, June 3-6, 2015. The omega-3 fatty acid metabolism in different Atlantic salmon families changes during the smoltification period Østbye, Tone-Kari K; Ruyter, Bente; Sonesson, Anna Kristina; Kjær, Marte Avranden; Baranski, Matthew; Bakke, Håvard; Thomassen, Magny Sissel S.; Sigholt, Trygve; Berge, Gerd Marit Nofima, P.O.Box 210, N-1431 Ås, Norway; bSalmo Breed AS, Bergen, Norway; cUniversity of Life Sciences, N-1431 Ås, Norway, dBioMar AS, Trondheim, Norway

199 J. Agric. Food Chem. 2015, 63, 4, 1261-1267 Publication Date:January 15, 2015 https://doi.org/10.1021/jf504863u Copyright © 2015 American Chemical Society

200 Baydas G, Gursu MF, Yilmaz S, et al. Daily rhythm of glutathione peroxidase activity, lipid peroxidation and glutathione levels in tissues of pinealectomized rats. Neurosci Lett. 2002;323(3):195–198. doi:10.1016/s0304-3940(02)00144-1

201 Díaz-Muñoz M, Hernández-Muñoz R, Suárez J, Chagoya de Sánchez V. Day-night cycle of lipid peroxidation in rat cerebral cortex and their relationship to the glutathione cycle and superoxide dismutase activity. Neuroscience. 1985;16(4):859–863. doi:10.1016/0306-4522(85)90100-9

202 Maciel, Fábio & Rosa, Carlos & Santos, EA & Monserrat, José & Nery, Luiz. (2004). Daily variations in oxygen consumption, antioxidant defenses, and lipid peroxidation in the gills and hepatopancreas of an estuarine crab. Canadian Journal of Zoology. 82. 10.1139/z04-182

203 Solar, Peter & Toth, G & Smajda, Benadik & Ahlers, I & Ahlersová, E. (1995). Circadian and circannual oscillations of tissue lipoperoxides in rats. Physiological research / Academia Scientiarum Bohemoslovaca. 44. 249-56

204 Bao, Ai-Min & Liu, Rong-Yu & Van Someren, Eus J W & Hofman, Michel A. & Cao, Yun-Xia & Zhou, Jiang-Ning. (2003). Diurnal rhythm of free estradiol during the menstrual cycle. European journal of endocrinology / European Federation of Endocrine Societies. 148. 227-32. 10.1530/eje.0.1480227

205 Díaz-Muñoz M, Hernández-Muñoz R, Suárez J, Chagoya de Sánchez V. Day-night cycle of lipid peroxidation in rat cerebral cortex and their relationship to the glutathione cycle and superoxide dismutase activity. Neuroscience. 1985;16(4):859–863. doi:10.1016/0306-4522(85)90100-9

206 Solár P, Ahlers I. Circadian oscillations of lipid peroxides in the rat pineal gland. Physiol Res. 1997;46(4):323–325

207 Moskovic DJ, Eisenberg ML, Lipshultz LI. Seasonal fluctuations in testosterone-estrogen ratio in men from the Southwest United States. J Androl. 2012;33(6):1298–1304. doi:10.2164/jandrol.112.016386

208 Demir A, Uslu M, Arslan OE. The effect of seasonal variation on sexual behaviors in males and its correlation with hormone levels: a prospective clinical trial. Cent European J Urol. 2016;69(3):285–289. doi:10.5173/ceju.2016.793

209 Kitson AP, Marks KA, Shaw B, Mutch DM, Stark KD. Treatment of ovariectomized rats with 17β-estradiol increases hepatic delta-6 desaturase enzyme expression and docosahexaenoic acid levels in hepatic and plasma phospholipids. Prostaglandins Leukot Essent Fatty Acids. 2013;89(2-3):81–88. doi:10.1016/j.plefa.2013.05.003

210 Ishihara Y, Itoh K, Tanaka M, et al. Potentiation of 17β-estradiol synthesis in the brain and elongation of seizure latency through dietary supplementation with docosahexaenoic acid. Sci Rep. 2017;7(1):6268. Published 2017 Jul 24. doi:10.1038/s41598-017-06630-0

211 Extier A, Perruchot MH, Baudry C, Guesnet P, Lavialle M, Alessandri JM. Differential effects of steroids on the synthesis of polyunsaturated fatty acids by human neuroblastoma cells. Neurochem Int. 2009;55(5):295–301. doi:10.1016/j.neuint.2009.03.009

212 Ruffoli R, Carpi A, Giambelluca MA, Grasso L, Scavuzzo MC, Giannessi F F. Diazepam administration prevents testosterone decrease and lipofuscin accumulation in testis of mouse exposed to chronic noise stress. Andrologia. 2006;38(5):159–165. doi:10.1111/j.1439-0272.2006.00732.x

213 Nagata C, Takatsuka N, Kawakami N, Shimizu H. Relationships between types of fat consumed and serum estrogen and androgen concentrations in Japanese men. Nutr Cancer. 2000;38(2):163–167. doi:10.1207/S15327914NC382_4

214 Marra CA, de Alaniz MJ. Influence of testosterone administration on the biosynthesis of unsaturated fatty acids in male and female rats. Lipids. 1989;24(12):1014–1019. doi:10.1007/bf02544071

215 Ves-Losada, A., Peluffo, R.O. Effect of L-triiodothyronine on Δ9 desaturase activity in liver microsomes of male rats. Lipids 24, 931–935 (1989). https://doi.org/10.1007/BF02544536

216 van Landeghem AA, Poortman J, Nabuurs M, Thijssen JH. Endogenous concentration and subcellular distribution of estrogens in normal and malignant human breast tissue. Cancer Res. 1985;45(6):2900–2906

217 Taniuchi S, Fujishima F, Miki Y, et al. Tissue concentrations of estrogens and aromatase immunolocalization in interstitial pneumonia of human lung. Mol Cell Endocrinol. 2014;392(1-2):136–143. doi:10.1016/j.mce.2014.05.016

218 Ikeda K, Shiraishi K, Yoshida A, Shinchi Y, Sanada M, Motooka Y, et al. (2016) Synchronous Multiple Lung Adenocarcinomas: Estrogen Concentration in Peripheral Lung. PLoS ONE 11(8): e0160910. https://doi.org/10.1371/journal.pone.0160910

219 Cortés-Gallegos V, Gallegos AJ, Basurto CS, Rivadeneyra J. Estrogen peripheral levels vs estrogen tissue concentration in the human female reproductive tract. J Steroid Biochem. 1975;6(1):15–20. doi:10.1016/0022-4731(75)90023-0

220 Vermeulen-Meiners C, Jaszmann LJ, Haspels AA, Poortman J, Thijssen JH. The endogenous concentration of estradiol and estrone in normal human postmenopausal endometrium. J Steroid Biochem. 1984;21(5):607–612. doi:10.1016/0022-4731(84)90338-8

221 Ishihara Y, Itoh K, Tanaka M, et al. Potentiation of 17β-estradiol synthesis in the brain and elongation of seizure latency through dietary supplementation with docosahexaenoic acid. Sci Rep. 2017;7(1):6268. Published 2017 Jul 24. doi:10.1038/s41598-017-06630-0

222 Tan NS, Frecer V, Lam TJ, Ding JL. Temperature dependence of estrogen binding: importance of a subzone in the ligand binding domain of a novel piscine estrogen receptor. Biochim Biophys Acta. 1999;1452(2):103–120. doi:10.1016/s0167-4889(99)00128-7

223 Panno ML, Sisci D, Salerno M, et al. Thyroid hormone modulates androgen and oestrogen receptor content in the Sertoli cells of peripubertal rats. J Endocrinol. 1996;148(1):43–50. doi:10.1677/joe.0.1480043

224 Olicina, G., Munoz, D., Kemp, J., Timon, R., Maynar, J., Caballero, M. & Maynar, M. (2012). Total plasma fatty acid responses to maximal incremental exercise after caffeine ingestion. Journal of Exercise Science and Fitness,10(1), 33-37. Retrieved from https://doi.org/10.1016/j.jesf.2012.04.008

225 Faas FH, Carter WJ. Fatty-acid desaturation and microsomal lipid fatty-acid composition in experimental hyperthyroidism. Biochem J. 1981;193(3):845–852. doi:10.1042/bj1930845

226 Liang T, Liao S. Inhibition of steroid 5 alpha-reductase by specific aliphatic unsaturated fatty acids. Biochem J. 1992;285 (Pt 2)(Pt 2):557–562. doi:10.1042/bj2850557

227 Takahashi, Mayumi & Tsuboyama-Kasaoka, Nobuyo & Nakatani, Teruyo & Ishii, Masami & Tsutsumi, Shuichi & Aburatani, Hiroyuki & Ezaki, Osamu. (2002). Fish oil feeding alters liver gene expressions to defend against PPAR?? activation and ROS production. American journal of physiology. Gastrointestinal and liver physiology. 282. G338-48. 10.1152/ajpgi.00376.2001

228 Calderon-Gierszal EL, Prins GS (2015) Directed Differentiation of Human Embryonic Stem Cells into Prostate Organoids In Vitro and its Perturbation by Low-Dose Bisphenol A Exposure. PLoS ONE 10(7): e0133238 https://doi.org/10.1371/journal.pone.0133238

229 Saffarini CM, McDonnell-Clark EV, Amin A, Huse SM, Boekelheide K. Developmental exposure to estrogen alters differentiation and epigenetic programming in a human fetal prostate xenograft model. PLoS One. 2015;10(3):e0122290. Published 2015 Mar 23. doi:10.1371/journal.pone.0122290

230 Frye CA, Edinger KL, Seliga AM, Wawrzycki JM. 5alpha-reduced androgens may have actions in the hippocampus to enhance cognitive performance of male rats. Psychoneuroendocrinology. 2004;29(8):1019–1027. doi:10.1016/j.psyneuen.2003.10.004

231 Edinger KL, Frye CA. Testosterone's anti-anxiety and analgesic effects may be due in part to actions of its 5alpha-reduced metabolites in the hippocampus. Psychoneuroendocrinology. 2005;30(5):418–430. doi:10.1016/j.psyneuen.2004.11.001

232 Jarvis TR, Chughtai B, Kaplan SA. Testosterone and benign prostatic hyperplasia. Asian J Androl 2015;17:212-6

233 Marks LS, Mazer NA, Mostaghel E, et al. Effect of Testosterone Replacement Therapy on Prostate Tissue in Men With Late-Onset Hypogonadism: A Randomized Controlled Trial. JAMA. 2006;296(19):2351–2361. doi:10.1001/jama.296.19.2351

234 Kjellman A, Akre O, Norming U, Törnblom M, Gustafsson O. Dihydrotestosterone levels and survival in screening-detected prostate cancer: a 15-yr follow-up study. Eur Urol. 2008;53(1):106–111. doi:10.1016/j.eururo.2007.04.063

235 Andersson SO, Baron J, Wolk A, Lindgren C, Bergström R, Adami HO. Early life risk factors for prostate cancer: a population-based case-control study in Sweden. Cancer Epidemiol Biomarkers Prev. 1995;4(3):187–192

236 Zhao Z, Reinstatler L, Klaassen Z, Xu Y, Yang X, Madi R, et al. (2016) The Association of Fatty Acid Levels and Gleason Grade among Men Undergoing Radical Prostatectomy. PLoS ONE 11(11): e0166594. https://doi.org/10.1371/journal.pone.0166594

237 Krieg M, Nass R, Tunn S. Effect of aging on endogenous level of 5 alpha-dihydrotestosterone, testosterone, estradiol, and estrone in epithelium and

stroma of normal and hyperplastic human prostate. J Clin Endocrinol Metab. 1993;77(2):375–381. doi:10.1210/jcem.77.2.7688377

238 Krieg M, Weisser H, Tunn S. Androgen- und Estrogenstoffwechsel in der menschlichen benignen Prostatahyperplasie (BPH) [Androgen and estrogen metabolism in human benign prostatic hyperplasia (BPH)]. Verh Dtsch Ges Pathol. 1993;77:19–24

239 Prins GS, Birch L, Habermann H, et al. Influence of neonatal estrogens on rat prostate development. Reprod Fertil Dev. 2001;13(4):241–252. doi:10.1071/rd00107

240 Kozák I, Bartsch W, Krieg M, Voigt KD. Nuclei of stroma: site of highest estrogen concentration in human benign prostatic hyperplasia. Prostate. 1982;3(5):433–438. doi:10.1002/pros.2990030503

241 Ishikawa T, Glidewell-Kenney C, Jameson JL. Aromatase-independent testosterone conversion into estrogenic steroids is inhibited by a 5 alpha-reductase inhibitor. J Steroid Biochem Mol Biol. 2006;98(2-3):133–138. doi:10.1016/j.jsbmb.2005.09.004

242 Sreeramulu D, Ramalakshmi BA, Balakrishna N, Raghuramulu N. Serum dehydroepiandrosterone and lipid peroxides in human volunteers of different age groups. Indian J Clin Biochem. 2004;19(1):79–82. doi:10.1007/BF02872396

243 Kaya H, Sezik M, Ozkaya O, Dittrich R, Siebzehnrubl E, Wildt L. Lipid peroxidation at various estradiol concentrations in human circulation during ovarian stimulation with exogenous gonadotropins. Horm Metab Res. 2004;36(10):693–695. doi:10.1055/s-2004-826018

244 Watanabe, Mayumi & Nakamura, Yoshinobu & Tomiyama, Chikako & Abo, Toru. (2016). A Specific Pattern in the Basal Body Temperature Chart during the First Week of Pregnancy May Warn of a Miscarriage Crisis. Health. 08. 723-729. 10.4236/health.2016.88075

245 Hinckley T Sr, Clark RM, Bushmich SL, Milvae RA. Long chain polyunsaturated fatty acids and bovine luteal cell function. Biol Reprod. 1996;55(2):445–449. doi:10.1095/biolreprod55.2.445

246 Robinson, Robert S & Pushpakumara, Anil & Cheng, Zhangrui & Peters, Andrew & Abayasekara, Dilkush & Wathes, D Claire. (2002). Effects of dietary polyunsaturated fatty acids on ovarian and uterine function in lactating dairy cows. Reproduction (Cambridge, England). 124. 119-31. 10.1530/rep.0.1240119.

247 Deol P, Evans JR, Dhahbi J, et al. Soybean Oil Is More Obesogenic and Diabetogenic than Coconut Oil and Fructose in Mouse: Potential Role for the Liver. PLoS One. 2015;10(7):e0132672. Published 2015 Jul 22. doi:10.1371/journal.pone.0132672

248 Lanna, Anna & Oliveira, Maria & Alves, Moreira. (2005). Effect of temperature on polyunsaturated fatty acid accumulation in soybean seeds. Brazilian Journal of Plant Physiology. 17. 10.1590/S1677-04202005000200004

249 Morrison, M.J. & Cober, E.R. & Saleem, M.F. & Mclaughlin, Neil & Frégeau Reid, Judith & Ma, B.L. & Woodrow, L.. (2010). Seasonal changes in temperature and precipitation influence isoflavone concentration in short-season soybean. Field Crops Research. 117. 113-121. 10.1016/j.fcr.2010.02.005

250 Cederroth CR, Zimmermann C, Nef S. Soy, phytoestrogens and their impact on reproductive health. Mol Cell Endocrinol. 2012;355(2):192–200. doi:10.1016/j.mce.2011.05.049

251 Effect of phytoestrogens on the endometrium? Foth, DoloresNawroth, Frank et al. Fertility and Sterility, Volume 83, Issue 1, 256 – 257

252 Hartley, D.E., Edwards, J.E., Spiller, C.E. et al. The soya isoflavone content of rat diet can increase anxiety and stress hormone release in the male rat. Psychopharmacology 167, 46–53 (2003). https://doi.org/10.1007/s00213-002-1369-7

253 Wood CE, Cline JM, Anthony MS, Register TC, Kaplan JR. Adrenocortical effects of oral estrogens and soy isoflavones in female monkeys. J Clin Endocrinol Metab. 2004;89(5):2319-2325. doi:10.1210/jc.2003-031728

254 Blasbalg TL, Hibbeln JR, Ramsden CE, Majchrzak SF, Rawlings RR. Changes in consumption of omega-3 and omega-6 fatty acids in the United States during the 20th century. Am J Clin Nutr. 2011;93(5):950–962. doi:10.3945/ajcn.110.006643

255 Siepmann T, Roofeh J, Kiefer FW, Edelson DG. Hypogonadism and erectile dysfunction associated with soy product consumption. Nutrition. 2011;27(7-8):859–862. doi:10.1016/j.nut.2010.10.018

256 Flegal KM, Carroll MD, Kuczmarski RJ, Johnson CL. Overweight and obesity in the United States: prevalence and trends, 1960-1994. Int J Obes Relat Metab Disord. 1998;22(1):39–47. doi:10.1038/sj.ijo.0800541

257 Tanaka M, Fujimoto K, Chihara Y, et al. Isoflavone supplements stimulated the production of serum equol and decreased the serum

dihydrotestosterone levels in healthy male volunteers. Prostate Cancer Prostatic Dis. 2009;12(3):247–252. doi:10.1038/pcan.2009.10

258 He C, Qu X, Wan J, Rong R, Huang L, Cai C, et al. (2012) Inhibiting Delta-6 Desaturase Activity Suppresses Tumor Growth in Mice. PLoS ONE 7(10): e47567. https://doi.org/10.1371/journal.pone.0047567

259 Powell DR, Gay JP, Smith M, et al. Fatty acid desaturase 1 knockout mice are lean with improved glycemic control and decreased development of atheromatous plaque. Diabetes, Metabolic Syndrome and Obesity: Targets and Therapy. 2016;9:185-199. doi:10.2147/DMSO.S106653

260 Yashiro H, Takagahara S, Tamura YO, Miyahisa I, Matsui J, Suzuki H, et al. (2016) A Novel Selective Inhibitor of Delta-5 Desaturase Lowers Insulin Resistance and Reduces Body Weight in Diet-Induced Obese C57BL/6J Mice. PLoS ONE 11(11): e0166198. https://doi.org/10.1371/journal. pone.0166198

261 Wahl HG, Kausch C, Machicao F, Rett K, Stumvoll M, Häring HU. Troglitazone downregulates delta-6 desaturase gene expression in human skeletal muscle cell cultures. Diabetes. 2002;51(4):1060–1065. doi:10.2337/ diabetes.51.4.1060

262 Mulligan CM, Le CH, deMooy AB, Nelson CB, Chicco AJ. Inhibition of delta-6 desaturase reverses cardiolipin remodeling and prevents contractile dysfunction in the aged mouse heart without altering mitochondrial respiratory function. J Gerontol A Biol Sci Med Sci. 2014;69(7):799–809. doi:10.1093/gerona/glt209

263 Gibson RA, Neumann MA, Lien EL, Boyd KA, Tu WC. Docosahexaenoic acid synthesis from alpha-linolenic acid is inhibited by diets high in polyunsaturated fatty acids. Prostaglandins Leukot Essent Fatty Acids. 2013;88(1):139–146. doi:10.1016/j.plefa.2012.04.003

264 Swenne, Ingemar & Vessby, Bengt. (2013). Relationship of Δ 6 -desaturase and Δ 5 -desaturase activities with thyroid hormone status in adolescents with eating disorders and weight loss. Acta paediatrica (Oslo, Norway : 1992). 102. 10.1111/apa.12132

265 Ves-Losada A, Peluffo RO. Effect of L-triiodothyronine on liver microsomal delta 6 and delta 5 desaturase activity of male rats. Mol Cell Biochem. 1993;121(2):149–153. doi:10.1007/bf00925974

266 Patel S, Paulsen C, Heffernan C, et al. Tuberculosis transmission in the Indigenous peoples of the Canadian prairies. PLoS One. 2017;12(11):e0188189. Published 2017 Nov 14. doi:10.1371/journal.pone.0188189

267 Bonilla DL, Fan YY, Chapkin RS, McMurray DN. Transgenic mice enriched in omega-3 fatty acids are more susceptible to pulmonary tuberculosis: impaired resistance to tuberculosis in fat-1 mice. J Infect Dis. 2010;201(3):399–408. doi:10.1086/650344

268 THE METABOLISM OF ESKIMOS. JAMA. 1929;92(10):808–809. doi:10.1001/jama.1929.02700360046013

269 Dubey P, Jayasooriya AP, Cheema SK. Diets Enriched in Fish-Oil or Seal-Oil have Distinct Effects on Lipid Levels and Peroxidation in BioF1B Hamsters. Nutr Metab Insights. 2011;4:7–17. Published 2011 Mar 23. doi:10.4137/NMI.S6728

270 Horrobin DF. Low prevalences of coronary heart disease (CHD), psoriasis, asthma and rheumatoid arthritis in Eskimos: are they caused by high dietary intake of eicosapentaenoic acid (EPA), a genetic variation of essential fatty acid (EFA) metabolism or a combination of both?. Med Hypotheses. 1987;22(4):421–428. doi:10.1016/0306-9877(87)90037-5

271 Drummond, Jack. "FATS IN THE LIFE OF THE NATION: CANTOR LECTURE." Journal of the Royal Society of Arts, vol. 96, no. 4775, 1948, pp. 569–581. JSTOR, www.jstor.org/stable/41363655. Accessed 7 Apr. 2020

272 Fodor JG, Helis E, Yazdekhasti N, Vohnout B. "Fishing" for the origins of the "Eskimos and heart disease" story: facts or wishful thinking?. Can J Cardiol. 2014;30(8):864–868. doi:10.1016/j.cjca.2014.04.007

273 Watkins JA. THE ALASKAN ESKIMO: THE PREVALENCE OF DISEASE AND THE SANITARY CONDITIONS OF THE VILLAGES ALONG THE ARCTIC COAST. Am J Public Health (N Y). 1914;4(8):643–648. doi:10.2105/ajph.4.8.643

274 Rabinowitch IM. Clinical and Other Observations on Canadian Eskimos in the Eastern Arctic. Can Med Assoc J. 1936;34(5):487–501

275 Bertelsen A. Grønlandsk medicinsk statistik og nosografi. Bd. III: Det sædvanlige grønlandske sygdomsbillede, [Medical statistics and nosography in Greenland: the usual disease pattern in Greenland], vol. 3. Meddelelser om Grønland 1940;117(3). From DET KONGELIGE INDUSTRI-, HANDVERK¬OG SKIPSFARTSDEPARTEMENT NORSK POLARINSTITUTT SKRIFTER Nr. 102 STUDIES ON THE BLOOD AND BLOOD PRESSURE IN THE ESKIMO AND THE SIGNIFICANCE OF KETOSIS UNDER ARCTIC CONDITIONS. I KOMMISJON HOS BRØGGERS BOKTRYKKERIS FORLAG OSLO 1954

276 Ho/ygaard, Arne. "Studies on the nutrition and physio-pathology of Eskimos." (1941).

277 BROWN GM, CRONK LB, BOAG TJ. The occurrence of cancer in an Eskimo. Cancer. 1952;5(1):142–143. doi:10.1002/1097-0142(195201)5:1<142::aid-cncr2820050119>3.0.co;2-q

278 Preliminary Survey of Dietary Intakes and Blood Levels of Cholesterol and the Occurrence of Cardiovascular Disease in the Eskimo. KARE RODAHL, Arctic Aeromedical Laboratory, Fairbanks, Alaska, and Institute of Physiology, Oslo University, Norway

279 GOTTMANN AW. A report of one hundred three autopsies on Alaskan natives. Arch Pathol. 1960;70:117–124

280 Lederman JM, Wallace AC & Hildes JA (1962): Arteriosclerosis andneoplasms in Canadian Eskimos. Biological aspect of aging. In:Proceedings of the Fifth International Congress on Gerontology. NewYork: Columbia University Press, pp 201 ± 207

281 DET KONGELIGE INDUSTRI-, HANDVERKOG SKIPSFARTSDEPARTEMENT NORSK POLARI N STITUTT. STUDIES ON THE BLOOD AND BLOOD PRESSURE IN THE ESKIMO AND THE SIGNIFICANCE OF KETOSIS UNDER ARCTIC CONDITIONS. I. K. Rodahl: 1954

282 Fortuine, R. (1969), Characteristics of cancer in the eskimos of Southwestern Alaska. Cancer, 23: 468–474. doi:10.1002/1097-0142(196902)23:2<468::AID-CNCR2820230225>3.0.CO;2-9

283 Mazess RB, Mather W. Bone mineral content of North Alaskan Eskimos. Am J Clin Nutr. 1974;27(9):916–925. doi:10.1093/ajcn/27.8.916

284 SCOTT EM, GRIFFITH IV, HOSKINS DD, WHALEY RD. Serum-cholesterol levels and blood-pressure of Alaskan Eskimo men. Lancet. 1958;2(7048):667–668. doi:10.1016/s0140-6736(58)92264-5

285 DAVIES LE, HANSON S. THE ESKIMOS OF THE NORTHWEST PASSAGE: A SURVEY OF DIETARY COMPOSITION AND VARIOUS BLOOD AND METABOLIC MEASUREMENTS. Can Med Assoc J. 1965;92(5):205–216

286 Bjerregaard P, Young TK, Hegele RA. Low incidence of cardiovascular disease among the Inuit--what is the evidence?. Atherosclerosis. 2003;166(2):351-357. doi:10.1016/s0021-9150(02)00364-7

287 ALASKA NATIVE HEALTH STATUS REPORT. Alaska Bureau of Vital Statistics http://anthctoday.org/epicenter/publications/HealthStatusReport/AN_HealthStatusReport_FINAL2017.pdf

288 FINAL REPORT ON THE ALASKA TRADITIONAL DIET SURVEY Prepared by Carol Ballew, Ph.D., Director Angela Ross, B.S., B.S., Research Coordinator Rebecca S. Wells, S.M., Epidemiologist Vanessa Hiratsuka, A.B., Public Health Educator Alaska Native Epidemiology Center Alaska Native Health Board 3700 Woodland Drive, Suite 500 Anchorage, AK 99517 907-562-6006 http://www.anhb.org In collaboration with Kari J. Hamrick, Ph.D., R.D. Senior Research Associate Institute for Circumpolar Health Studies University of Alaska Anchorage. FINAL REPORT ON THE ALASKA TRADITIONAL DIET SURVEY Prepared by Carol Ballew

289 Sven O. E. Ebbesson, Patricia M. Risica, Lars O. E. Ebbesson & John M. Kennish (2005) Eskimos have CHD despite high consumption of omega-3 fatty acids: the Alaska Siberia project, International Journal of Circumpolar Health, 64:4, 387-395, DOI: 10.3402/ijch.v64i4.18015

290 Schæbel LH, Vestergaard H, Laurberg P, Rathcke CN, Andersen S. Intake of traditional Inuit diet vary in parallel with inflammation as estimated from YKL-40 and hsCRP in Inuit and non-Inuit in Greenland. Atherosclerosis. 2013;228(2):496–501. doi:10.1016/j.atherosclerosis.2013.03.022

291 Ebbesson, Sven & Roman, Mary & Devereux, Richard & Kaufman, David & Fabsitz, Richard & Maccluer, Jean & Dyke, Bennett & Laston, Sandra & Wenger, Charlotte & Comuzzie, Anthony & Romenesko, Terry & Ebbesson, Lars & Nobmann, E & Howard, Barbara. (2008). Consumption of omega-3 fatty acids is not associated with a reduction in carotid atherosclerosis: The Genetics of Coronary Artery Disease in Alaska Natives study. Atherosclerosis. 199. 346-353. 10.1016/j.atherosclerosis.2007.10.020.

292 Cutchins A, Roman MJ, Devereux RB, et al. Prevalence and correlates of subclinical atherosclerosis in Alaska Eskimos: the GOCADAN study. Stroke. 2008;39(11):3079–3082. doi:10.1161/STROKEAHA.108.519199

293 Ostergaard Kristensen M. Increased incidence of bleeding intracranial aneurysms in Greenlandic Eskimos. Acta Neurochir (Wien). 1983;67(1-2):37–43. doi:10.1007/bf01401666

294 Alkerwi A, Shivappa N, Crichton G, Hébert JR. No significant independent relationships with cardiometabolic biomarkers were detected in the Observation of Cardiovascular Risk Factors in Luxembourg

study population. Nutr Res. 2014;34(12):1058–1065. doi:10.1016/j.nutres.2014.07.017

295 Stark KD, Van Elswyk ME, Higgins MR, Weatherford CA, Salem N Jr. Global survey of the omega-3 fatty acids, docosahexaenoic acid and eicosapentaenoic acid in the blood stream of healthy adults. Prog Lipid Res. 2016;63:132–152. doi:10.1016/j.plipres.2016.05.001

296 Micha, Renata et al. "Global, regional, and national consumption levels of dietary fats and oils in 1990 and 2010: a systematic analysis including 266 country-specific nutrition surveys." BMJ (2014). BMJ 2014;348:g2272

297 Nick Townsend, Lauren Wilson, Prachi Bhatnagar, Kremlin Wickramasinghe, Mike Rayner, Melanie Nichols, Cardiovascular disease in Europe: epidemiological update 2016, European Heart Journal, Volume 37, Issue 42, 7 November 2016, Pages 3232–3245, https://doi.org/10.1093/eurheartj/ehw334

298 Grundy SM. What is the desirable ratio of saturated, polyunsaturated, and monounsaturated fatty acids in the diet?. Am J Clin Nutr. 1997;66(4 Suppl):988S–990S. doi:10.1093/ajcn/66.4.988S

299 Eilander A, Harika RK, Zock PL. Intake and sources of dietary fatty acids in Europe: Are current population intakes of fats aligned with dietary recommendations?. Eur J Lipid Sci Technol. 2015;117(9):1370–1377. doi:10.1002/ejlt.201400513

300 Eilander A, Harika RK, Zock PL. Intake and sources of dietary fatty acids in Europe: Are current population intakes of fats aligned with dietary recommendations?. Eur J Lipid Sci Technol. 2015;117(9):1370–1377. doi:10.1002/ejlt.201400513

301 Townsend N, Wilson L, Bhatnagar P, Wickramasinghe K, Rayner M, Nichols M. Cardiovascular disease in Europe: epidemiological update 2016 [published correction appears in Eur Heart J. 2019 Jan 7;40(2):189]. Eur Heart J. 2016;37(42):3232–3245. doi:10.1093/eurheartj/ehw334

302 Gersten, Omer & Wilmoth, John. (2002). The Cancer Transition in Japan since 1951. Demographic Research. 7. 271-306. 10.4054/DemRes.2002.7.5

303 Sekikawa A, Miyamoto Y, Miura K, et al. Continuous decline in mortality from coronary heart disease in Japan despite a continuous and marked rise in total cholesterol: Japanese experience after the Seven Countries Study. Int J Epidemiol. 2015;44(5):1614–1624. doi:10.1093/ije/dyv143

304 Turin TC, Okuda N, Miura K, et al. Iron Intake and Associated Factors in General Japanese Population: NIPPON DATA80, NIPPON DATA90 and

National Nutrition Monitoring. Journal of Epidemiology. 2010;20(Suppl 3):S557-S566. doi:10.2188/jea.JE20090225

305 Cook, J.D. & Morck, Timothy & Lynch, Sean. (1982). The inhibitory effect of soy products on non-heme iron absorption in man. The American journal of clinical nutrition. 34. 2622-9. 10.1093/ajcn/34.12.2622

306 Willcox DC, Scapagnini G, Willcox BJ. Healthy aging diets other than the Mediterranean: a focus on the Okinawan diet. Mech Ageing Dev. 2014;136-137:148–162. doi:10.1016/j.mad.2014.01.002

307 Nakamura, Yasuyuki & Ueshima, Hirotsugu & Okamura, Tomonori & Kadowaki, Takashi & Hayakawa, Takehito & Kita, Yoshikuni & Tamaki, Shinji & Okayama, Akira. (2005). Association between fish consumption and all-cause and cause-specific mortality in Japan: NIPPON DATA80, 1980–99. The American journal of medicine. 118. 239-45. 10.1016/j.amjmed.2004.12.016

308 Ito Y, Shimizu H, Yoshimura T, et al. Serum concentrations of carotenoids, alpha-tocopherol, fatty acids, and lipid peroxides among Japanese in Japan, and Japanese and Caucasians in the US. Int J Vitam Nutr Res. 1999;69(6):385–395. doi:10.1024/0300-9831.69.6.385

309 Rylander C, Sandanger TM, Engeset D, Lund E (2014) Consumption of Lean Fish Reduces the Risk of Type 2 Diabetes Mellitus: A Prospective Population Based Cohort Study of Norwegian Women. PLoS ONE 9(2): e89845 https://doi.org/10.1371/journal.pone.0089845

310 Crombie IK, McLoone P, Smith WC, Thomson M, Pedoe HT. International differences in coronary heart disease mortality and consumption of fish and other foodstuffs. Eur Heart J. 1987;8(6):560–563. doi:10.1093/oxfordjournals.eurheartj.a062322

311 Hibbeln JR, Nieminen LR, Blasbalg TL, Riggs JA, Lands WE. Healthy intakes of n-3 and n-6 fatty acids: estimations considering worldwide diversity. Am J Clin Nutr. 2006;83(6 Suppl):1483S–1493S. doi:10.1093/ajcn/83.6.1483S

312 Bjorgvinsdottir L, Arnar DO, Indridason OS, et al. Do high levels of n-3 polyunsaturated fatty acids in cell membranes increase the risk of postoperative atrial fibrillation?. Cardiology. 2013;126(2):107–114. doi:10.1159/000351432

313 https://ec.europa.eu/fisheries/6-consumption_en

314 Gunnarsdottir I, Gustavsdottir AG, Thorsdottir I. Iodine intake and status in Iceland through a period of 60 years. Food Nutr Res. 2009;53:10.3402/fnr.v53i0.1925. Published 2009 May 27. doi:10.3402/fnr.v53i0.1925

315 Skuladottir GV, Heidarsdottir R, Arnar DO, et al. Plasma n-3 and n-6 fatty acids and the incidence of atrial fibrillation following coronary artery bypass graft surgery. Eur J Clin Invest. 2011;41(9):995-1003. doi:10.1111/j.1365-2362.2011.02497.x

316 Schaich, K.M. 2014. Lipid co-oxidation of proteins: One size does not fit all. Inform, 25(3): 134-139

317 Beaudoin-Chabot C, Wang L, Smarun AV, Vidović D, Shchepinov MS and Thibault G (2019) Deuterated Polyunsaturated Fatty Acids Reduce Oxidative Stress and Extend the Lifespan of C. elegans. Front. Physiol. 10:641. doi: 10.3389/fphys.2019.00641

318 Gómez-Cortés P, Sacks GL, Brenna JT. Quantitative analysis of volatiles in edible oils following accelerated oxidation using broad spectrum isotope standards. Food Chem. 2015;174:310–318. doi:10.1016/j.foodchem.2014.11.015

319 Yang KM, Cheng MC, Chen CW, Tseng CY, Lin LY, Chiang PY. Characterization of Volatile Compounds with HS-SPME from Oxidized n-3 PUFA Rich Oils via Rancimat Tests. J Oleo Sci. 2017;66(2):113–122. doi:10.5650/jos.ess16157

320 Pilar Gómez-Cortés, Gavin L. Sacks, J. Thomas Brenna, Quantitative analysis of volatiles in edible oils following accelerated oxidation using broad spectrum isotope standards, Food Chemistry, Volume 174, 2015, Pages 310-318, ISSN 0308-8146, https://doi.org/10.1016/j.foodchem.2014.11.015. (http://www.sciencedirect.com/science/article/pii/S0308814614017440)

321 Ohta T, Iijima K, Miyamoto M, et al. Loss of Keap1 function activates Nrf2 and provides advantages for lung cancer cell growth. Cancer Res. 2008;68(5):1303–1309. doi:10.1158/0008-5472.CAN-07-5003

322 Chenere P. Ramsey, Charles A. Glass, Marshall B. Montgomery, Kathryn A. Lindl, Gillian P. Ritson, Luis A. Chia, Ronald L. Hamilton, Charleen T. Chu, Kelly L. Jordan-Sciutto; Expression of Nrf2 in Neurodegenerative Diseases, Journal of Neuropathology & Experimental Neurology, Volume 66, Issue 1, 1 January 2007, Pages 75–85, https://doi.org/10.1097/nen.0b013e31802d6da9

323 Ni M, Li X, Yin Z, et al. Methylmercury induces acute oxidative stress, altering Nrf2 protein level in primary microglial cells. Toxicol Sci. 2010;116(2):590-603

324 Lewis KN, Wason E, Edrey YH, Kristan DM, Nevo E, Buffenstein R. Regulation of Nrf2 signaling and longevity in naturally long-lived rodents. Proc Natl Acad Sci U S A. 2015;112(12):3722-7

325 Zhang H, Davies KJA, Forman HJ. Oxidative stress response and Nrf2 signaling in aging. Free Radic Biol Med. 2015;88(Pt B):314-336. YU, T. & DAY, EDGAR & SINNHUBER, RUSSELL. (2006). Autoxidation of Fish Oils. I. Identification of Volatile Monocarbonyl Compounds from Autoxidized Salmon Oil b, c. Journal of Food Science. 26. 192 - 197. 10.1111/j.1365-2621.1961.tb00791.x

326 J. Crilly, Matthew & D. Tryon, Liam & T. Erlich, Avigail & Hood, David. (2016). The role of Nrf2 in skeletal muscle contractile and mitochondrial function. Journal of Applied Physiology. 121. jap.00042.2016. 10.1152/japplphysiol.00042.2016

327 Takahashi, Mayumi & Tsuboyama-Kasaoka, Nobuyo & Nakatani, Teruyo & Ishii, Masami & Tsutsumi, Shuichi & Aburatani, Hiroyuki & Ezaki, Osamu. (2002). Fish oil feeding alters liver gene expressions to defend against PPAR?? activation and ROS production. American journal of physiology. Gastrointestinal and liver physiology. 282. G338-48. 10.1152/ajpgi.00376.2001

328 D'Aquino M, Benedetti PC, Di Felice M, et al. Effect of fish oil and coconut oil on antioxidant defence system and lipid peroxidation in rat liver. Free Radic Res Commun. 1991;12-13 Pt 1:147–152. doi:10.3109/10715769109145779

329 Yip PK, Pizzasegola C, Gladman S, Biggio ML, Marino M, Jayasinghe M, et al. (2013) The Omega-3 Fatty Acid Eicosapentaenoic Acid Accelerates Disease Progression in a Model of Amyotrophic Lateral Sclerosis. PLoS ONE 8(4): e61626. https://doi.org/10.1371/journal.pone.0061626

330 Labuschagne CF, van den Broek NJF, Postma P, Berger R, Brenkman AB (2013) A Protocol for Quantifying Lipid Peroxidation in Cellular Systems by F2-Isoprostane Analysis. PLoS ONE 8(11): e80935 https://doi.org/10.1371/journal.pone.0080935

331 331, T. & DAY, EDGAR & SINNHUBER, RUSSELL. (2006). Autoxidation of Fish Oils. I. Identification of Volatile Monocarbonyl Compounds from Autoxidized Salmon Oil b, c. Journal of Food Science. 26. 192 - 197. 10.1111/j.1365-2621.1961.tb00791.x

332 WYATT, C. & DAY, E.. (2006). Autoxidation of Fish Oils. II. Changes in the Carbonyl Distribution of Autoxidizing Salmon Oils b. Journal of Food Science. 28. 305 - 312. 10.1111/j.1365-2621.1963.tb00202.x

333 Ritter JC, Budge SM. Key lipid oxidation products can be used to predict sensory quality of fish oils with different levels of EPA and DHA. Lipids. 2012;47(12):1169–1179. doi:10.1007/s11745-012-3733-7, Frankel EN (2005) Lipid oxidation, 2nd edn. The Oily Press, Bridgwater

334 WYATT, C. & DAY, E.. (2006). Autoxidation of Fish Oils. II. Changes in the Carbonyl Distribution of Autoxidizing Salmon Oils b. Journal of Food Science. 28. 305 - 312. 10.1111/j.1365-2621.1963.tb00202.x.

335 YU, T. & DAY, EDGAR & SINNHUBER, RUSSELL. (2006). Autoxidation of Fish Oils. I. Identification of Volatile Monocarbonyl Compounds from Autoxidized Salmon Oil b, c. Journal of Food Science. 26. 192 - 197. 10.1111/j.1365-2621.1961.tb00791.x

336 Lee, H. & Kizito, S.A. & Weese, S.J. & Craig-Schmidt, M.C. & Lee, Y. & Wei, C.-I & An, H.. (2006). Analysis of Headspace Volatile and Oxidized Volatile Compounds in DHA-enriched Fish Oil on Accelerated Oxidative Storage. Journal of Food Science. 68. 2169 - 2177. 10.1111/j.1365-2621.2003.tb05742.x.

337 Cameron-Smith D, Albert BB, Cutfield WS. Fishing for answers: is oxidation of fish oil supplements a problem? Journal of Nutritional Science. 2015;4:e36. doi:10.1017/jns.2015.26

338 Petersen DR, Saba LM, Sayin VI, Papagiannakopoulos T, Schmidt EE, Merrill GF, et al. (2018) Elevated Nrf-2 responses are insufficient to mitigate protein carbonylation in hepatospecific PTEN deletion mice. PLoS ONE 13(5): e0198139. https://doi.org/10.1371/journal.pone.0198139

339 Casañas-Sánchez V, Pérez JA, Fabelo N, Quinto-Alemany D and Díaz ML (2015) Docosahexaenoic (DHA) modulates phospholipid-hydroperoxide glutathione peroxidase (Gpx4) gene expression to ensure self-protection from oxidative damage in hippocampal cells. Front. Physiol. 6:203. doi: 10.3389/fphys.2015.00203

340 Parola M, Barrera G, Carasso MC, et al. Variazioni delle attivita' adenosintrifosfatasiche in plasma membrane incubate "in vitro" in presenza di 4-idrossi-2,3-nonenale [Changes in the adenosinetriphosphatase activity in plasma membranes incubated in vitro in the presence of 4-hydroxy-2,3-nonenal]. Boll Soc Ital Biol Sper. 1982;58(18):1199–1205

341 Van Kuijk FJ, Holte LL, Dratz EA. 4-Hydroxyhexenal: a lipid peroxidation product derived from oxidized docosahexaenoic acid. Biochim Biophys Acta. 1990;1043(1):116–118. doi:10.1016/0005-2760(90)90118-h

342 Yamada S, Funada T, Shibata N, et al. Protein-bound 4-hydroxy-2-hexenal as a marker of oxidized n-3 polyunsaturated fatty acids. J Lipid Res. 2004;45(4):626–634. doi:1

343 Kapusta A, Kuczyńska B, Puppel K (2018) Relationship between the degree of antioxidant protection and the level of malondialdehyde in high-performance Polish Holstein-Friesian cows in peak of lactation. PLoS ONE 13(3): e0193512. https://doi.org/10.1371/journal.pone.0193512

344 Alves Luzia L, Mendes Aldrighi J, Teixeira Damasceno NR, et al. FISH OIL AND VITAMIN E CHANGE LIPID PROFILES AND ANTI-LDL-ANTIBODIES IN TWO DIFFERENT ETHNIC GROUPS OF WOMEN TRANSITIONING THROUGH MENOPAUSE. Nutr Hosp. 2015;32(1):165–174. Published 2015 Jul 1. doi:10.3305/nh.2015.32.1.9079

345 Nair PP, Judd JT, Berlin E, et al. Dietary fish oil-induced changes in the distribution of alpha-tocopherol, retinol, and beta-carotene in plasma, red blood cells, and platelets: modulation by vitamin E. Am J Clin Nutr. 1993;58(1):98–102. doi:10.1093/ajcn/58.1.98

346 Haglund O, Luostarinen R, Wallin R, Wibell L, Saldeen T. The effects of fish oil on triglycerides, cholesterol, fibrinogen and malondialdehyde in humans supplemented with vitamin E. J Nutr. 1991;121(2):165–169. doi:10.1093/jn/121.2.165

347 Filaire E, Massart A, Portier H, et al. Effect of 6 Weeks of n-3 fatty-acid supplementation on oxidative stress in Judo athletes. Int J Sport Nutr Exerc Metab. 2010;20(6):496–506. doi:10.1123/ijsnem.20.6.496

348 Allard JP, Kurian R, Aghdassi E, Muggli R, Royall D. Lipid peroxidation during n-3 fatty acid and vitamin E supplementation in humans. Lipids. 1997;32(5):535–541. doi:10.1007/s11745-997-0068-2

349 Gaweł, Stefan & Wardas, Maria & Niedworok, Elzbieta & Wardas, Piotr. (2004). [Malondialdehyde (MDA) as a lipid peroxidation marker]. Wiadomości lekarskie (Warsaw, Poland : 1960). 57. 453-5.

350 Gil P, Fariñas F, Casado A, López-Fernández E. Malondialdehyde: a possible marker of ageing. Gerontology. 2002;48(4):209–214. doi:10.1159/000058352

351 Kapusta A, Kuczyńska B, Puppel K (2018) Relationship between the degree of antioxidant protection and the level of malondialdehyde in

high-performance Polish Holstein-Friesian cows in peak of lactation. PLoS ONE 13(3): e0193512. https://doi.org/10.1371/journal.pone.0193512

352 Shibata A, Uemura M, Hosokawa M, Miyashita K. Acrolein as a Major Volatile in the Early Stages of Fish Oil TAG Oxidation. J Oleo Sci. 2018;67(5):515–524. doi:10.5650/jos.ess17235

353 Shibata, Ako & Uemura, Mariko & Hosokawa, Masashi & Miyashita, Kazuo. (2015). Formation of Acrolein in the Autoxidation of Triacylglycerols with Different Fatty Acid Compositions. Journal of the American Oil Chemists' Society. 92. 10.1007/s11746-015-2732-2

354 The Possible Carcinogenicity of Overcooked Meats, Heated Cholesterol, Acrolein, and Heated Sesame Oil Paul E. Steiner, Robert Steele and F. C. Koch Cancer Res February 1 1943 (3) (2) 100-107

355 Uchida, Koji & Kanematsu, Masamichi & Kensuke, Sakai & Matsuda, Tsukasa & Hattori, Nobutaka & Mizuno, Yoshikuni & Suzuki, Daisuke & Miyata, Toshio & Noguchi, Noriko & Niki, Etsuo & Osawa, Toshihiko. (1998). Protein-bound acrolein: Potential markers for oxidative stress. Proceedings of the National Academy of Sciences of the United States of America. 95. 4882-7. 10.1073/pnas.95.9.4882

356 Hochman DJ, Collaco CR, Brooks EG. Acrolein induction of oxidative stress and degranulation in mast cells. Environ Toxicol. 2014;29(8):908–915. doi:10.1002/tox.21818

357 Yang Y, Zhang Z, Zhang H, et al. Effects of maternal acrolein exposure during pregnancy on testicular testosterone production in fetal rats. Mol Med Rep. 2017;16(1):491–498. doi:10.3892/mmr.2017.6624

358 Tomitori H, Usui T, Saeki N, et al. Polyamine oxidase and acrolein as novel biochemical markers for diagnosis of cerebral stroke. Stroke. 2005;36(12):2609–2613. doi:10.1161/01.STR.0000190004.36793.2d

359 Depner CM, Traber MG, Bobe G, Kensicki E, Bohren KM, et al. (2013) A Metabolomic Analysis of Omega-3 Fatty Acid-Mediated Attenuation of Western Diet-Induced Nonalcoholic Steatohepatitis in LDLR-/- Mice. PLoS ONE 8(12): e83756. doi:10.1371/journal.pone.0083756

360 Depner CM, Traber MG, Bobe G, Kensicki E, Bohren KM, et al. (2013) A Metabolomic Analysis of Omega-3 Fatty Acid-Mediated Attenuation of Western Diet-Induced Nonalcoholic Steatohepatitis in LDLR-/- Mice. PLoS ONE 8(12): e83756. doi:10.1371/journal.pone.0083756

361 Miller E, Morel A, Saso L, Saluk J. Isoprostanes and neuroprostanes as biomarkers of oxidative stress in neurodegenerative diseases. Oxid Med Cell Longev. 2014;2014:572491. doi:10.1155/2014/572491

362 Yin, Huiyong & Musiek, Erik & Gao, Ling & Porter, Ned & Morrow, Jason. (2005). Regiochemistry of Neuroprostanes Generated from the Peroxidation of Docosahexaenoic Acid. The Journal of biological chemistry. 280. 26600-11. 10.1074/jbc.M503088200

363 Reich EE, Markesbery WR, Roberts LJ 2nd, Swift LL, Morrow JD, Montine TJ. Brain regional quantification of F-ring and D-/E-ring isoprostanes and neuroprostanes in Alzheimer's disease. Am J Pathol. 2001;158(1):293–297. doi:10.1016/S0002-9440(10)63968-5

364 Cecarini V, Ding Q, Keller JN. Oxidative inactivation of the proteasome in Alzheimer's disease. Free Radic Res. 2007;41(6):673–680. doi:10.1080/10715760701286159

365 Signorini C, De Felice C, Durand T, et al. Relevance of 4-F4t-neuroprostane and 10-F4t-neuroprostane to neurological diseases. Free Radic Biol Med. 2018;115:278–287. doi:10.1016/j.freeradbiomed.2017.12.009

366 Rodríguez-Lagunas MJ, Ferrer R, Moreno JJ. Effect of eicosapentaenoic acid-derived prostaglandin E3 on intestinal epithelial barrier function. Prostaglandins Leukot Essent Fatty Acids. 2013;88(5):339–345. doi:10.1016/j.plefa.2013.02.001

367 SCIENTISTS AND THEIR SPECIALTIES Beltsville. Human Nutrition Research Center. W.Mertz,Director. Beltsville Agricultural Research Center-East Beltsville, Maryland, 20705. SPRING 1987

368 Dobrian AD, Lieb DC, Cole BK, Taylor-Fishwick DA, Chakrabarti SK, Nadler JL. Functional and pathological roles of the 12- and 15-lipoxygenases. Prog Lipid Res. 2011;50(1):115–131. doi:10.1016/j.plipres.2010.10.005

369 Dobrian AD, Lieb DC, Cole BK, Taylor-Fishwick DA, Chakrabarti SK, Nadler JL. Functional and pathological roles of the 12- and 15-lipoxygenases. Prog Lipid Res. 2011;50(1):115–131. doi:10.1016/j.plipres.2010.10.005

370 Ambaw, Y.A., Chao, C., Ji, S. et al. Tear eicosanoids in healthy people and ocular surface disease. Sci Rep 8, 11296 (2018). https://doi.org/10.1038/s41598-018-29568-3

371 Nordøy A, Hatcher L, Goodnight S, Fitzgerald GA, Conner WE. Effects of dietary fat content, saturated fatty acids, and fish oil on eicosanoid production and hemostatic parameters in normal men. J Lab Clin Med. 1994;123(6):914–920

372 Palmer SM, Robinson LJ, Wang A, Gossage JR, Bashore T, Tapson VF. Massive pulmonary edema and death after prostacyclin infusion in a patient with pulmonary veno-occlusive disease. Chest. 1998;113(1):237–240. doi:10.1378/chest.113.1.237

373 Harrison JL, Rowe RK, Ellis TW, et al. Resolvins AT-D1 and E1 differentially impact functional outcome, post-traumatic sleep, and microglial activation following diffuse brain injury in the mouse. Brain Behav Immun. 2015;47:131–140. doi:10.1016/j.bbi.2015.01.001

374 DeBlois, E. T. 1882. The origin of the menhaden industry. Bull. U.S. Fish Comm. 1 : 46-51

375 ASTRACK, A., SORBYE, O., BRASCH, A. and HUBER, W. (1952), EFFECTS OF HIGH INTENSITY ELECTRON BURSTS UPON VARIOUS VEGETABLE AND FISH OILSa. Journal of Food Science, 17: 571-583. doi:10.1111/j.1365-2621.1952.tb16802.x

376 376 Vol. 17, No. 2 FEBRUARY 1955 FISH and WILDLIFE SERVICE United States Department of the Interior Washington DC

377 MARCH 1958. FISH and WILDLIFE SERVICE. United States Department of the Interior Washington, D.C UNITED STATES. DEPARTMENT OF THE INTERIOR

378 June 1958 COMMERCIAL FISHERIES REVIEW. Vol. 20, No.6 parentheses (p) is added by author

379 Commercial Fisheries Review vol .17 no.3 march 1955

380 COMMERCIAL FISHERIES REVIEW Vol. 20, No.6. June 1958

381 COMMERCIAL FISHERIES REVIEW . Vol . 21, No.1. January 1959

382 Utilization of FATS in Poultry and Other Livestock Feeds. 1960. Utilization Research Report No. 2 UNITED STATES DEPARTMENT OF AGRICULTURE. Agricultural Research Service August 1960

383 Nutritive value of marine oils. 1. Menhaden oil at varying oxidation levels, with and without antioxidants in rat diets. Author(s) : ASHEED, A. A.; OLDFIELD, J. E.; KAUFMES, J.; SINNHUBER, R. O. Author Affiliation : Dept. Animal Sci., Oregon State Univ., Corvallis. Journal article : Journal of Nutrition 1963 Vol.79 pp.323-332

384 Lin CF, Asghar A, Gray JI, et al. Effects of oxidised dietary oil and antioxidant supplementation on broiler growth and meat stability. Br Poult Sci. 1989;30(4):855–864. doi:10.1080/00071668908417212

385 April 1957 - Supplement COMMERCIAL FISHERIES REVIEW 11. FEEDING FISH OILS TO DOMESTIC ANIMALS By J. E. Oldfield, * Allen F. Anglemier; * and M. E. Stansby

386 July 1958 COMMERCIAL FISHERIES REVIEW vol.20 nr.7

387 Commercial Fisheries Review, Volume 21, April, No. 1, 1959

388 commericial fisheries review 1958 july vol. 20 no. 7.

389 Vol. 17, No. 2 FEBRUARY 1955 Commercial Fisheries Review

390 Commercial Fisheries Review. April 1958. Vol. 20, No. 4

391 Commercial Fisheries ReviewVol.17,No.9 SEPTEMBER 1955

392 Venolia, A.W. and Tappel, A.L. (1958), Brown-colored oxypolymers of unsaturated fats. J Am Oil Chem Soc, 35: 135-138. doi:10.1007/BF02640596

393 Benjamin H. Ershoff, Effects of Diet on Fish Oil Toxicity in the Rat, The Journal of Nutrition, Volume 71, Issue 1, May 1960, Pages 45–53, https://doi.org/10.1093/jn/71.1.45

394 Flanagan - Int, 2879 UNITED STATES FISH AND WILDLIFE SERVICE For Release AUGUST 17, 1958

395 July 1958 COMMERCIAL FISHERIES REVIEW vol.20 nr.7

396 PEIFER JJ, JANSSEN F, AHN P, COX W, LUNDBERG WO. Studies on the distribution of lipides in hypercholesteremic rats. I. The effect of feeding palmitate, oleate, linoleate, linolenate, menhaden and tuna oils. Arch Biochem Biophys. 1960;86:302–308. doi:10.1016/0003-9861(60)90422-7

397 Commercial Fisheries Review. Vol. 22, No.7 July 1960

398 Commercial Fisheries Review. July 1958. Vol 20. No. 7

399 Determination of Peroxide Values for Rancidity in Fish Oils. Maurice Stansby. Ind. Eng. Chem. Anal. Ed., 1941, 13 (9), pp 627–631 DOI: 10.1021/i560097a017 Publication Date: September 1941

400 Federal Fishery Research in the Pacific Northwest Preceding Formation of Northwest Fisheries Center, U.S . DEPARTMENT OF COMMERCE. National Oceanic and Atmospheric Administration National Marine Fisheries Service. Maurice E. Stansby November 1979

401 GOEBEL, C. Ueber Pigmentablagerung in der Darmmusculatur. Virchow Arch Path Anat z36:482-522, I894

402 György P, Goldblatt H. OBSERVATIONS ON THE CONDITIONS OF DIETARY HEPATIC INJURY (NECROSIS, CIRRHOSIS) IN RATS. J Exp Med. 1942;75(4):355–368. doi:10.1084/jem.75.4.355

403 Heidary F, Vaeze Mahdavi MR, Momeni F, Minaii B, Rogani M, Fallah N, et al. (2008) Food Inequality Negatively Impacts Cardiac Health in Rabbits. PLoS ONE 3(11): e3705. https://doi.org/10.1371/journal.pone.0003705

404 WOOD EM, YASUTAKE WT. Ceroid in fish. Am J Pathol. 1956;32(3):591–603

405 Nutritional study of ageing. 4. Effect of fish oil on the appearance of ceroid pigment in rats. KOYANAGI, T.; FURUKAWA, R.; MIYASHI, K. Journal article : Journal of Japanese Society of Food and Nutrition 1969Vol.22pp.148-151. Martin L. Katz, Holly J. Stientjes, Chun-Lan Gao, and J. Scott Christianson

406 THE IN VITRO PREPARATION AND HISTOCHEMICAL PROPERTIES OF SUBSTANCES RESEMBLING CEROID* BY W. G. BRUCE CASSELMAN,$ M.D. (From the Banting and Best Department of Medical Research, University of Toronto, Toronto, Canada) PLATE 39 (Received for publication, August 4, 1951

407 CEROID" PIGMENT IN HUMAN TISSUES * ALwIN M. PAPPENHEIMER, M.D.,t and JOSEPH VICTOR, M.D. (From the Department of Pathology, College of Physicians and Surgeons, Columbia University, and from the First Division, Research Service, Goldwater Memorwl Hospital, New York, N. Y.)1945

408 Nye SW, Chittayasothorn K. Ceroid in the gastrointestinal smooth muscle of the Thai-Lao ethnic group. Am J Pathol. 1967;51(2):287–299

409 Perše M, Injac R, Erman A (2013) Oxidative Status and Lipofuscin Accumulation in Urothelial Cells of Bladder in Aging Mice. PLoS ONE 8(3): e59638. https://doi.org/10.1371/journal.pone.0059638

410 Perše M, Injac R, Erman A (2013) Oxidative Status and Lipofuscin Accumulation in Urothelial Cells of Bladder in Aging Mice. PLoS ONE 8(3): e59638. https://doi.org/10.1371/journal.pone.0059638 This author doesn't think that for example the heart cells are post-miotic. Anversa P, Kajstura J, Leri A, Bolli R. Life and death of cardiac stem cells: a paradigm shift in cardiac biology. Circulation. 2006;113(11):1451–1463. doi:10.1161/CIRCULATIONAHA.105.595181

411 Markelic, Milica & Velickovic, Ksenija & Golic, Igor & Klepal, Waltraud & Otasevic, Vesna & Stancic, Ana & Jankovic, Aleksandra & Vucetic, Milica & Buzadzic, Biljana & Korac, Bato & Korac, Aleksandra. (2013). The origin of lipofuscin in brown adipocytes of hyperinsulinaemic rats: The role of

lipid peroxidation and iron. Histology and histopathology. 28. 10.14670/HH-28.493

412 Brizzee, K.R., Eddy, D.E., Harman, D. et al. Free radical theory of aging: Effect of dietary lipids on lipofuscin accumulation in the hippocampus of rats. AGE 7, 9–15 (1984). https://doi.org/10.1007/BF02431889

413 Harris C. A lipofuscin-like pigment in the kidneys of estrogen-treated rats. Arch Pathol. 1966;82(4):353–355

414 Brunk, Ulf & Terman, Alexei. (2002). The mitochondrial-lysosomal axis theory of aging. European Journal of Biochemistry. 269. 1996-2002. 10.1046/j.1432-1033.2002.02869.x

415 Baixauli F, Acín-Pérez R, Villarroya-Beltrí C, et al. Mitochondrial Respiration Controls Lysosomal Function during Inflammatory T Cell Responses. Cell Metab. 2015;22(3):485–498. doi:10.1016/j.cmet.2015.07.020

416 Terman A, Brunk UT. The aging myocardium: roles of mitochondrial damage and lysosomal degradation. Heart Lung Circ. 2005;14(2):107–114. doi:10.1016/j.hlc.2004.12.023

417 Iqbal M, Dingle JT, Moore T, Sharman IM. Nutrition and lysosomal activity. The effect of dietary cod-liver oil on the distribution of polyunsaturated fatty acids in the kidney lysosomes of rats receiving deficient or adequate intakes of vitamin E. Br J Nutr. 1969;23(1):31–39. doi:10.1079/bjn19690006

418 Flood JF, Morley PM, Morley JE. Age-related changes in learning, memory, and lipofuscin as a function of the percentage of SAMP8 genes. Physiol Behav. 1995;58(4):819–822. doi:10.1016/0031-9384(95)00125-3

419 Kumar, P., Taha, A., Sharma, D. et al. Effect of dehydroepiandrosterone (DHEA) on monoamine oxidase activity, lipid peroxidation and lipofuscin accumulation in aging rat brain regions. Biogerontology 9, 235–246 (2008). https://doi.org/10.1007/s10522-008-9133-y

420 Kumar, P., Taha, A., Sharma, D. et al. Effect of dehydroepiandrosterone (DHEA) on monoamine oxidase activity, lipid peroxidation and lipofuscin accumulation in aging rat brain regions. Biogerontology 9, 235–246 (2008). https://doi.org/10.1007/s10522-008-9133-y

421 Hsu, C.-Y. and Chiu, Y.-C. (2009), Ambient temperature influences aging in an annual fish (Nothobranchius rachovii). Aging Cell, 8: 726-737. doi:10.1111/j.1474-9726.2009.00525.x

422 GORHAM JR, BOE N, BAKER GA. Experimental "yellow fat" disease in pigs. Cornell Vet. 1951;41(4):332–338

423 MASON KE, DAM H, GRANADOS H. Histological changes in adipose tissue of rats fed a vitamin E deficient diet high in cod liver oil. Anat Rec. 1946;94:265–287. doi:10.1002/ar.1090940305

424 Canadian Journal of Comparative Medicine Steatitis 1 Alberta Mink Vol. XXIl, NO. 7 July, 1956

425 Danse LH, Steenbergen-Botterweg WA. Early changes of yellow fat disease in mink fed a vitamin-E deficient diet supplemented with fresh or oxidised fish oil. Zentralbl Veterinarmed A. 1976;23(8):645–660. doi:10.1111/j.1439-0442.1976.tb01530.x

426 Hendriks HR, Eestermans IL. Phagocytosis and lipofuscin accumulation in lymph node macrophages. Mech Ageing Dev. 1986;35(2):161–167. doi:10.1016/0047-6374(86)90006-0

427 Solfrizzi V, D'Introno A, Colacicco AM, et al. Unsaturated fatty acids intake and all-causes mortality: a 8.5-year follow-up of the Italian Longitudinal Study on Aging. Exp Gerontol. 2005;40(4):335–343. doi:10.1016/j. exger.2005.01.003

428 Hulbert AJ, Faulks SC, Harper JM, Miller RA, Buffenstein R. Extended longevity of wild-derived mice is associated with peroxidation-resistant membranes. Mech Ageing Dev. 2006;127(8):653–657. doi:10.1016/j. mad.2006.03.002

429 Valencak TG, Ruf T. N-3 polyunsaturated fatty acids impair lifespan but have no role for metabolism. Aging Cell. 2007;6(1):15–25. doi:10.1111/j.1474-9726.2006.00257.x

430 Hulbert AJ, Pamplona R, Buffenstein R, Buttemer WA. Life and death: metabolic rate, membrane composition, and life span of animals. Physiol Rev. 2007;87(4):1175–1213. doi:10.1152/physrev.00047.2006

431 Jové M, Naudí A, Aledo JC, et al. Plasma long-chain free fatty acids predict mammalian longevity. Sci Rep. 2013;3:3346. Published 2013 Nov 28. doi:10.1038/srep03346

432 Genetic and Chemical Effects on Somatic and Germline Aging Volume 2019 |Article ID 5768953 / https://doi.org/10.1155/2019/5768953 The Effects of Age and Reproduction on the Lipidome of Caenorhabditis elegans Qin-Li Wan,1 Zhong-Lin Yang, Xiao-Gang Zhou, Ai-Jun Ding, Yuan-Zhu Pu,1 Huai-Rong Luo and Gui-Sheng Wu

433 Collino S, Montoliu I, Martin F-PJ, Scherer M, Mari D, Salvioli S, et al. (2013) Metabolic Signatures of Extreme Longevity in Northern Italian Centenarians Reveal a Complex Remodeling of Lipids, Amino Acids,

and Gut Microbiota Metabolism. PLoS ONE 8(3): e56564. https://doi.org/10.1371/journal.pone.0056564

434 Pamplona R, Portero-Otín M, Ruiz C, Gredilla R, Herrero A, Barja G. Double bond content of phospholipids and lipid peroxidation negatively correlate with maximum longevity in the heart of mammals. Mech Ageing Dev. 2000;112(3):169–183. doi:10.1016/s0047-6374(99)00045-7

435 Spindler SR, Mote PL, Flegal JM. Dietary supplementation with Lovaza and krill oil shortens the life span of long-lived F1 mice. Age (Dordr). 2014;36(3):9659. doi:10.1007/s11357-014-9659-7

436 López-Domínguez JA, Ramsey JJ, Tran D, et al. The Influence of Dietary Fat Source on Life Span in Calorie Restricted Mice. J Gerontol A Biol Sci Med Sci. 2015;70(10):1181–1188. doi:10.1093/gerona/glu177

437 Strong R, Miller RA, Antebi A, et al. Longer lifespan in male mice treated with a weakly estrogenic agonist, an antioxidant, an α-glucosidase inhibitor or a Nrf2-inducer. Aging Cell. 2016;15(5):872–884. doi:10.1111/acel.12496

438 Collino S, Montoliu I, Martin F-PJ, Scherer M, Mari D, Salvioli S, et al. (2013) Metabolic Signatures of Extreme Longevity in Northern Italian Centenarians Reveal a Complex Remodeling of Lipids, Amino Acids, and Gut Microbiota Metabolism. PLoS ONE 8(3): e56564. https://doi.org/10.1371/journal.pone.0056564

439 Page RE Jr, Peng CY. Aging and development in social insects with emphasis on the honey bee, Apis mellifera L. Exp Gerontol. 2001;36(4-6):695–711. doi:10.1016/s0531-5565(00)00236-9

440 Mao W, Schuler MA, Berenbaum MR. A dietary phytochemical alters caste-associated gene expression in honey bees. Sci Adv. 2015;1(7):e1500795. Published 2015 Aug 28. doi:10.1126/sciadv.1500795

441 Asencot, Moshe & Lensky, Yaacov. (1988). The effect of soluble sugars in stored royal jelly on the differentiation of female honeybee (Apis mellifera L.) larvae to queens. Insect Biochemistry. 18. 127-133. 10.1016/0020-1790(88)90016-9

442 Haddad LS, Kelbert L, Hulbert AJ. Extended longevity of queen honey bees compared to workers is associated with peroxidation-resistant membranes. Exp Gerontol. 2007;42(7):601–609. doi:10.1016/j.exger.2007.02.008

443 Mitchell TW, Buffenstein R, Hulbert AJ. Membrane phospholipid composition may contribute to exceptional longevity of the naked mole-rat (Heterocephalus glaber): a comparative study using shotgun lipidomics. Exp Gerontol. 2007;42(11):1053–1062. doi:10.1016/j.exger.2007.09.004

444 Kaufman AE, Verma JN, Goldfine H. Disappearance of plasmalogen-containing phospholipids in Megasphaera elsdenii. J Bacteriol. 1988;170(6):2770-2774. doi:10.1128/jb.170.6.2770-2774.1988

445 Munro D, Blier PU. The extreme longevity of Arctica islandica is associated with increased peroxidation resistance in mitochondrial membranes. Aging Cell. 2012;11(5):845–855. doi:10.1111/j.1474-9726.2012.00847.x

446 Kujoth GC, Bradshaw PC, Haroon S, Prolla TA (2007) The Role of Mitochondrial DNA Mutations in Mammalian Aging. PLoS Genet 3(2): e24. https://doi.org/10.1371/journal.pgen.0030024

447 Portero-Otín M, Bellmunt MJ, Ruiz MC, Barja G, Pamplona R. Correlation of fatty acid unsaturation of the major liver mitochondrial phospholipid classes in mammals to their maximum life span potential. Lipids. 2001;36(5):491–498. doi:10.1007/s11745-001-0748-y

448 Pamplona R, Portero-Otín M, Riba D, et al. Mitochondrial membrane peroxidizability index is inversely related to maximum life span in mammals. J Lipid Res. 1998;39(10):1989–1994

449 Arranz L, Naudí A, De la Fuente M, Pamplona R. Exceptionally old mice are highly resistant to lipoxidation-derived molecular damage. Age (Dordr). 2013;35(3):621–635. doi:10.1007/s11357-012-9391-0

450 Pirke KM, Doerr P. Age related changes in free plasma testosterone, dihydrotestosterone and oestradiol. Acta Endocrinol (Copenh). 1975;80(1):171–178. doi:10.1530/acta.0.0800171

451 Puca AA, Andrew P, Novelli V, et al. Fatty acid profile of erythrocyte membranes as possible biomarker of longevity. Rejuvenation Res. 2008;11(1):63–72. doi:10.1089/rej.2007.0566

452 Schmidt S, Willers J, Riecker S, Möller K, Schuchardt JP, Hahn A. Effect of omega-3 polyunsaturated fatty acids on the cytoskeleton: an open-label intervention study. Lipids Health Dis. 2015;14:4. Published 2015 Feb 14. doi:10.1186/1476-511X-14-4

453 Harbige LS. Fatty acids, the immune response, and autoimmunity: a question of n-6 essentiality and the balance between n-6 and n-3. Lipids. 2003;38(4):323–341. doi:10.1007/s11745-003-1067-z

454 Han SN, Wu D, Ha WK, et al. Vitamin E supplementation increases T helper 1 cytokine production in old mice infected with influenza virus. Immunology. 2000;100(4):487–493. doi:10.1046/j.1365-2567.2000.00070.x

455 Wallace FA, Miles EA, Evans C, Stock TE, Yaqoob P, Calder PC. Dietary fatty acids influence the production of Th1- but not Th2-type cytokines. J Leukoc Biol. 2001;69(3):449–457

456 Kaasgaard SG, Hølmer G, Høy CE, Behrens WA, Beare-Rogers JL. Effects of dietary linseed oil and marine oil on lipid peroxidation in monkey liver in vivo and in vitro. Lipids. 1992;27(10):740–745. doi:10.1007/bf02535843

457 MOORE T, SHARMAN IM. Prevention of the injurious effects of excessive cod-liver oil by its fortification with vitamin E. Br J Nutr. 1961;15:297–303. doi:10.1079/bjn19610035

458 Meydani, S.N., Shapiro, A.C., Meydani, M. et al. Effect of age and dietary fat (fish, corn and coconut oils) on tocopherol status of C57BL/6Nia mice. Lipids 22, 345–350 (1987). https://doi.org/10.1007/BF02534004

459 Wolf G. The discovery of the antioxidant function of vitamin E: the contribution of Henry A. Mattill. J Nutr. 2005;135(3):363–366. doi:10.1093/jn/135.3.363

460 Steatitis on Mink Farms in Alberta. G. S. Wilton, Canadian Journal of Comparati" Modicime Steatiis 1 Alberta Mink Vol. XXIl, NO. 7. July, 1958

461 Das NP. Effects of vitamin A and its analogs on nonenzymatic lipid peroxidation in rat brain mitochondria. J Neurochem. 1989;52(2):585–588. doi:10.1111/j.1471-4159.1989.tb09159.x

462 H. A. Mattill, Calvin Golumbic, Vitamin E, Cod Liver Oil and Muscular Dystrophy: One Figure, The Journal of Nutrition, Volume 23, Issue 6, June 1942, Pages 625–631, https://doi.org/10.1093/jn/23.6.625

463 Nickels JD, Chatterjee S, Stanley CB, Qian S, Cheng X, Myles DAA, et al. (2017) The in vivo structure of biological membranes and evidence for lipid domains. PLoS Biol 15(5): e2002214. https://doi.org/10.1371/journal.pbio.2002214

464 Zhao W, Tian Y, Cai M, Wang F, Wu J, Gao J, et al. (2014) Studying the Nucleated Mammalian Cell Membrane by Single Molecule Approaches. PLoS ONE 9(5): e91595. https://doi.org/10.1371/journal.pone.0091595

465 Valentine RC, Valentine DL. Omega-3 fatty acids in cellular membranes: a unified concept. Prog Lipid Res. 2004;43(5):383–402. doi:10.1016/j.plipres.2004.05.004

466 Zhao W, Tian Y, Cai M, Wang F, Wu J, Gao J, et al. (2014) Studying the Nucleated Mammalian Cell Membrane by Single Molecule Approaches. PLoS ONE 9(5): e91595. https://doi.org/10.1371/journal.pone.0091595

467 Zhao W, Tian Y, Cai M, Wang F, Wu J, Gao J, et al. (2014) Studying the Nucleated Mammalian Cell Membrane by Single Molecule Approaches. PLoS ONE 9(5): e91595. https://doi.org/10.1371/journal.pone.0091595

468 Brenner RR. Effect of unsaturated acids on membrane structure and enzyme kinetics. Prog Lipid Res. 1984;23(2):69–96. doi:10.1016/0163-7827(84)90008-0

469 Ralph T. Holman. Autoxidation of fats and related substances. Progress in the Chemistry of Fats and other Lipids 1954, 2, 51-98. DOI: 10.1016/0079-6832(54)90004-X.

470 Hoch FL. Lipids and thyroid hormones. Prog Lipid Res. 1988;27(3):199–270. doi:10.1016/0163-7827(88)90013-6. Permission from Elsevier

471 Gorria M, Tekpli X, Sergent O, et al. Membrane fluidity changes are associated with benzo[a]pyrene-induced apoptosis in F258 cells: protection by exogenous cholesterol. Ann N Y Acad Sci. 2006;1090:108–112. doi:10.1196/annals.1378.011

472 Antunes-Madeira, M.D.C., Almeida, L.M. and Madeira, V.M.C. (1991), DDT-membrane interactions studied with two fluorescent probes. Pestic. Sci., 33: 347-357. doi:10.1002/ps.2780330308

473 Yilmaz B, Sandal S, Chen CH, Carpenter DO. Effects of PCB 52 and PCB 77 on cell viability, [Ca(2+)](i) levels and membrane fluidity in mouse thymocytes. Toxicology. 2006;217(2-3):184–193. doi:10.1016/j.tox.2005.09.008

474 Sarkar SN, Balasubramanian SV, Sikdar SK. Effect of fenvalerate, a pyrethroid insecticide on membrane fluidity. Biochimica et Biophysica Acta. 1993 Apr;1147(1):137-142. DOI: 10.1016/0005-2736(93)90324-s.

475 Sok M, Sentjurc M, Schara M, Stare J, Rott T. Cell membrane fluidity and prognosis of lung cancer. Ann Thorac Surg. 2002;73(5):1567–1571. doi:10.1016/s0003-4975(02)03458-6

476 Increased plasma membrane fluidity and decreased receptor availability of nonmuscle cells in myotonic dystrophy. C. Hübner, S.G. Lindner, M. Albani, M. Ballmann, B. Keup, M. Schürmann, H. Stegner, M. Claussen

477 Dave JR, Witorsch RJ. Prolactin increases lipid fluidity and prolactin binding of rat prostatic membranes. Am J Physiol. 1985;248(6 Pt 1):E687–E693. doi:10.1152/ajpendo.1985.248.6.E687

478 Tsuda K, Kimura K, Nishio I, Masuyama Y. Nitric oxide improves membrane fluidity of erythrocytes in essential hypertension: An electron paramagnetic resonance investigation. Biochem Biophys Res Commun. 2000;275(3):946–954. doi:10.1006/bbrc.2000.3408

479 Tsuda, Kazushi and Ichiro Nishio. "Role of estrogens in the regulation of membrane microviscosity." Circulation research 94 2 (2004): e17

480 Owada T, Miyashita Y, Motomura T, Onishi M, Yamashita S, Yamamoto N. Enhancement of human immunodeficiency virus type 1 (HIV-1) infection via increased membrane fluidity by a cationic polymer. Microbiol Immunol. 1998;42(2):97–107. doi:10.1111/j.1348-0421.1998.tb02257.x

481 Evani SJ, Ramasubramanian AK. Biophysical regulation of Chlamydia pneumoniae-infected monocyte recruitment to atherosclerotic foci. Sci Rep. 2016;6:19058. Published 2016 Jan 20. doi:10.1038/srep19058

482 Collins JM, Scott RB, McClish DK, Taylor JR, Grogan WM. Altered membrane anisotropy gradients of plasma membranes of living peripheral blood leukocytes in aging and Alzheimer's disease. Mech Ageing Dev. 1991;59(1-2):153–162. doi:10.1016/0047-6374(91)90081-a

483 Usami M, Komurasaki T, Hanada A, Kinoshita K, Ohata A. Effect of gamma-linolenic acid or docosahexaenoic acid on tight junction permeability in intestinal monolayer cells and their mechanism by protein kinase C activation and/or eicosanoid formation. Nutrition. 2003;19(2):150–156. doi:10.1016/s0899-9007(02)00927-9

484 Usami M, Komurasaki T, Hanada A, Kinoshita K, Ohata A. Effect of gamma-linolenic acid or docosahexaenoic acid on tight junction permeability in intestinal monolayer cells and their mechanism by protein kinase C activation and/or eicosanoid formation. Nutrition. 2003;19(2):150–156. doi:10.1016/s0899-9007(02)00927-9

485 Yafang, Ma & Zhou, G.H. & Li, Yingqiu & Zhu, Yingying & Yu, Xiaobo & Zhao, Fan & Li, He & Xu, Xing-Lian & Li, Chunbao. (2018). Intake of Fish Oil Specifically Modulates Colonic Muc2 Expression in Middle-Aged Rats by Suppressing the Glycosylation Process. Molecular Nutrition & Food Research. 62. 10.1002/mnfr.201700661.

486 van Hees NJM, Giltay EJ, Geleijnse JM, Janssen N, van der Does W (2014) DHA Serum Levels Were Significantly Higher in Celiac Disease Patients Compared to Healthy Controls and Were Unrelated to Depression. PLoS ONE 9(5): e97778. https://doi.org/10.1371/journal.pone.0097778

487 García JJ, Reiter RJ, Guerrero JM, et al. Melatonin prevents changes in microsomal membrane fluidity during induced lipid peroxidation. FEBS Lett. 1997;408(3):297–300. doi:10.1016/s0014-5793(97)00447-x

488 Choe M, Jackson C, Yu BP. Lipid peroxidation contributes to age-related membrane rigidity. Free Radic Biol Med. 1995;18(6):977–984. doi:10.1016/0891-5849(94)00217-8

489 Bonilla DL, Ly LH, Fan Y-Y, Chapkin RS, McMurray DN (2010) Incorporation of a Dietary Omega 3 Fatty Acid Impairs Murine Macrophage Responses to Mycobacterium tuberculosis. PLoS ONE 5(5): e10878. https://doi.org/10.1371/journal.pone.0010878

490 Pompéia C., Lopes L.R., Miyasaka C.K., Procópio J., Sannomiya P., Curi R.. Effect of fatty acids on leukocyte function. Braz J Med Biol Res [Internet]. 2000 Nov [cited 2020 Feb 25] ; 33(11): 1255-1268. Available from: http://www.scielo.br/scielo.php?script=sci_arttext&pid=S0100-879X2000001100001&lng=en. https://doi.org/10.1590/S0100-879X2000001100001

491 Meydani SN, Lichtenstein AH, Cornwall S, et al. Immunologic effects of national cholesterol education panel step-2 diets with and without fish-derived N-3 fatty acid enrichment. J Clin Invest. 1993;92(1):105–113. doi:10.1172/JCI116537

492 Kelley VE, Kirkman RL, Bastos M, Barrett LV, Strom TB. Enhancement of immunosuppression by substitution of fish oil for olive oil as a vehicle for cyclosporine. Transplantation. 1989;48(1):98–102. doi:10.1097/00007890-198907000-00023

493 Robinson DR, Prickett JD, Polisson R, Steinberg AD, Levine L. The protective effect of dietary fish oil on murine lupus. Prostaglandins. 1985;30(1):51–75. doi:10.1016/s0090-6980(85)80010-1

494 Diaz, Olivier & Berquand, Alexandre & Dubois, Madeleine & Agostino, Silvia & Sette, Claudio & Bourgoin, Sylvain & Lagarde, Michel & Nemoz, Georges & Prigent, Annie-France. (2002). The Mechanism of Docosahexaenoic Acid-induced Phospholipase D Activation in Human Lymphocytes Involves Exclusion of the Enzyme from Lipid Rafts. The Journal of biological chemistry. 277. 39368-78. 10.1074/jbc.M202376200

495 Vida C, de Toda IM, Cruces J, Garrido A, Gonzalez-Sanchez M, De la Fuente M. Role of macrophages in age-related oxidative stress and lipofuscin accumulation in mice. Redox Biol. 2017;12:423–437. doi:10.1016/j.redox.2017.03.005

496 Chow SC, Jondal M. Polyunsaturated free fatty acids stimulate an increase in cytosolic Ca2+ by mobilizing the inositol 1,4,5-trisphosphate-sensitive

Ca2+ pool in T cells through a mechanism independent of phosphoinositide turnover. J Biol Chem. 1990;265(2):902–907

497 Erickson KL, Hubbard NE. Dietary fish oil modulation of macrophage tumoricidal activity. Nutrition. 1996;12(1 Suppl):S34–S38. doi:10.1016/0899-9007(96)90016-7

498 van der Poll T, Marchant A, Buurman WA, et al. Endogenous IL-10 protects mice from death during septic peritonitis. J Immunol. 1995;155(11):5397–5401

499 Couper KN, Blount DG, Riley EM. IL-10: the master regulator of immunity to infection. J Immunol. 2008;180(9):5771–5777. doi:10.4049/jimmunol.180.9.5771

500 Brombacher TM, Nono JK, De Gouveia KS, et al. IL-13-Mediated Regulation of Learning and Memory. J Immunol. 2017;198(7):2681–2688. doi:10.4049/jimmunol.1601546

501 Gadani SP, Cronk JC, Norris GT, Kipnis J. IL-4 in the brain: a cytokine to remember. J Immunol. 2012;189(9):4213–4219. doi:10.4049/jimmunol.1202246

502 Moradkhani S, Jafarzadeh A, Bazargan-Harandi N, Baneshi MR, Mohammadi MM. Association of reduced count of interleukin-13-producing cells in breast milk with atopic dermatitis in infancy. Indian J Med Res. 2018;148(3):317–322. doi:10.4103/ijmr.IJMR_1682_16

503 Krauss-Etschmann S, Hartl D, Rzehak P, et al. Decreased cord blood IL-4, IL-13, and CCR4 and increased TGF-beta levels after fish oil supplementation of pregnant women. J Allergy Clin Immunol. 2008;121(2):464–470.e6. doi:10.1016/j.jaci.2007.09.018

504 Robert Irons, Kevin L. Fritsche, Omega-3 Polyunsaturated Fatty Acids Impair In Vivo Interferon-γ Responsiveness via Diminished Receptor Signaling, The Journal of Infectious Diseases, Volume 191, Issue 3, 1 February 2005, Pages 481– 486, https://doi.org/10.1086/427264

505 Rockett BD, Franklin A, Harris M, Teague H, Rockett A, Shaikh SR. Membrane raft organization is more sensitive to disruption by (n-3) PUFA than nonraft organization in EL4 and B cells. J Nutr. 2011;141(6):1041–1048. doi:10.3945/jn.111.138750

506 Pickering AM, Lehr M, Miller RA. Lifespan of mice and primates correlates with immunoproteasome expression. J Clin Invest. 2015;125(5):2059–2068. doi:10.1172/JCI80514

507 Sooksawate T, Simmonds MA. Effects of membrane cholesterol on the sensitivity of the GABA(A) receptor to GABA in acutely dissociated rat hippocampal neurones. Neuropharmacology. 2001;40(2):178–184. doi:10.1016/s0028-3908(00)00159-3

508 de la Torre MC, Torán P, Serra-Prat M, et al. Serum levels of immunoglobulins and severity of community-acquired pneumonia. BMJ Open Respir Res. 2016;3(1):e000152. Published 2016 Nov 28. doi:10.1136/bmjresp-2016-000152

509 James J. Pestka, Hui-Ren Zhou, Qunshan Jia, Ann M. Timmer, Dietary Fish Oil Suppresses Experimental Immunoglobulin A Nephropathy in Mice, The Journal of Nutrition, Volume 132, Issue 2, February 2002, Pages 261–269, https://doi.org/10.1093/jn/132.2.261

510 Snel J, Born L, van der Meer R. Dietary fish oil impairs induction of gamma-interferon and delayed-type hypersensitivity during a systemic Salmonella enteritidis infection in rats. APMIS. 2010;118(8):578–584. doi:10.1111/j.1600-0463.2010.02630.x

511 Diepersloot RJ, Bouter KP, Beyer WE, Hoekstra JB, Masurel N. Humoral immune response and delayed type hypersensitivity to influenza vaccine in patients with diabetes mellitus. Diabetologia. 1987;30(6):397–401. doi:10.1007/bf00292541

512 Christou NV, Meakins JL, Gordon J, et al. The delayed hypersensitivity response and host resistance in surgical patients. 20 years later. Ann Surg. 1995;222(4):534–548. doi:10.1097/00000658-199522240-00011

513 Teague H, Harris M, Whelan J, Comstock SS, Fenton JI, Shaikh SR. Short-term consumption of n-3 PUFAs increases murine IL-5 levels, but IL-5 is not the mechanistic link between n-3 fatty acids and changes in B-cell populations. J Nutr Biochem. 2016;28:30–36. doi:10.1016/j.jnutbio.2015.09.012

514 Reiman RM, Thompson RW, Feng CG, et al. Interleukin-5 (IL-5) augments the progression of liver fibrosis by regulating IL-13 activity. Infect Immun. 2006;74(3):1471–1479. doi:10.1128/IAI.74.3.1471-1479.2006

515 Fernandes G, Bysani C, Venkatraman JT, Tomar V, Zhao W. Increased TGF-beta and decreased oncogene expression by omega-3 fatty acids in the spleen delays onset of autoimmune disease in B/W mice. J Immunol. 1994;152(12):5979–5987

516 Meng XM, Nikolic-Paterson DJ, Lan HY. TGF-β: the master regulator of fibrosis. Nat Rev Nephrol. 2016;12(6):325–338. doi:10.1038/nrneph.2016.48

517 Alonso-Merino E, Martín Orozco R, Ruíz-Llorente L, et al. Thyroid hormones inhibit TGF-β signaling and attenuate fibrotic responses. Proc Natl Acad Sci U S A. 2016;113(24):E3451–E3460. doi:10.1073/pnas.1506113113

518 Krauss-Etschmann S, Hartl D, Rzehak P, et al. Decreased cord blood IL-4, IL-13, and CCR4 and increased TGF-beta levels after fish oil supplementation of pregnant women. J Allergy Clin Immunol. 2008;121(2):464–470.e6. doi:10.1016/j.jaci.2007.09.018

519 Chang HR, Arsenijevic D, Vladoianu IR, Girardier L, Dulloo AG. Fish oil enhances macrophage tumor necrosis factor-alpha mRNA expression at the transcriptional level. Metabolism. 1995;44(6):800–805. doi:10.1016/0026-0495(95)90196-5

520 Chang HR, Arsenijevic D, Pechère JC, et al. Dietary supplementation with fish oil enhances in vivo synthesis of tumor necrosis factor. Immunol Lett. 1992;34(1):13–17. doi:10.1016/0165-2478(92)90021-f

521 Virella G, Fourspring K, Hyman B, et al. Immunosuppressive effects of fish oil in normal human volunteers: correlation with the in vitro effects of eicosapentanoic acid on human lymphocytes. Clin Immunol Immunopathol. 1991;61(2 Pt 1):161–176. doi:10.1016/s0090-1229(05)80021-2

522 Bechoua S, Dubois M, Véricel E, Chapuy P, Lagarde M, Prigent AF. Influence of very low dietary intake of marine oil on some functional aspects of immune cells in healthy elderly people. Br J Nutr. 2003;89(4):523–531. doi:10.1079/BJN2002805

523 Metabolism. 1992 Jan;41(1):1-2. Fish oil decreases natural resistance of mice to infection with Salmonella typhimurium. Chang HR1, Dulloo AG, Vladoianu IR, Piguet PF, Arsenijevic D, Girardier L, Pechère JC

524 Woodworth HL, McCaskey SJ, Duriancik DM, et al. Dietary fish oil alters T lymphocyte cell populations and exacerbates disease in a mouse model of inflammatory colitis. Cancer Res. 2010;70(20):7960–7969. doi:10.1158/0008-5472.CAN-10-1396

525 Schwerbrock NMJ, Karlsson EA, Shi Q, Sheridan PA, Beck MA. Fish Oil-Fed Mice Have Impaired Resistance to Influenza Infection. The Journal of Nutrition. 2009;139(8):1588-1594. doi:10.3945/jn.109.108027

526 Shaikh SR, Edidin M. Polyunsaturated fatty acids and membrane organization: elucidating mechanisms to balance immunotherapy and susceptibility to infection. Chem Phys Lipids. 2008;153(1):24–33. doi:10.1016/j.chemphyslip.2008.02.008

527 Ghosh, Sanjoy & Decoffe, Daniella & Brown, Kirsty & Rajendiran, Ethendhar & Estaki, Mehrbod & Dai, Ben & Yip, Ashley & Gibson, Deanna. (2013). Fish Oil Attenuates Omega-6 Polyunsaturated Fatty Acid-Induced Dysbiosis and Infectious Colitis but Impairs LPS Dephosphorylation Activity Causing Sepsis. PloS one. 8. e55468. 10.1371/journal.pone.0055468

528 Yaqoob P, Calder P. Effects of dietary lipid manipulation upon inflammatory mediator production by murine macrophages. Cell Immunol. 1995;163(1):120–128. doi:10.1006/cimm.1995.1106

529 Irons R, Anderson MJ, Zhang M, Fritsche KL. Dietary fish oil impairs primary host resistance against Listeria monocytogenes more than the immunological memory response. J Nutr. 2003;133(4):1163–1169. doi:10.1093/jn/133.4.1163

530 Bechoua S, Dubois M, Véricel E, Chapuy P, Lagarde M, Prigent AF. Influence of very low dietary intake of marine oil on some functional aspects of immune cells in healthy elderly people. Br J Nutr. 2003;89(4):523–531. doi:10.1079/BJN2002805

531 van der Heide JJ, Bilo HJ, Donker JM, Wilmink JM, Tegzess AM. Effect of dietary fish oil on renal function and rejection in cyclosporine-treated recipients of renal transplants. N Engl J Med. 1993;329(11):769–773. doi:10.1056/NEJM199309093291105

532 Hashimoto M, Shinozuka K, Gamoh S, et al. The hypotensive effect of docosahexaenoic acid is associated with the enhanced release of ATP from the caudal artery of aged rats. J Nutr. 1999;129(1):70–76. doi:10.1093/jn/129.1.70

533 Cauwels, A., Rogge, E., Vandendriessche, B. et al. Extracellular ATP drives systemic inflammation, tissue damage and mortality. Cell Death Dis 5, e1102 (2014). https://doi.org/10.1038/cddis.2014.70

534 M Rossato, M Merico, A Bettella, P Bordon, C Foresta, Extracellular ATP stimulates estradiol secretion in rat Sertoli cells in vitro: modulation by external sodium, Molecular and Cellular Endocrinology, Volume 178, Issues 1–2, 2001, Pages 181-187, ISSN 0303-7207, https://doi.org/10.1016/S0303-7207(01)00426-9. (http://www.sciencedirect.com/science/article/pii/S0303720701004269)

535 Nuñez L, Villalobos C, Frawley LS. Extracellular ATP as an autocrine/paracrine regulator of prolactin release. Am J Physiol. 1997;272(6 Pt 1):E1117–E1123. doi:10.1152/ajpendo.1997.272.6.E1117

536 Inscho EW, Belott TP, Mason MJ, Smith JB, Navar LG. Extracellular ATP increases cytosolic calcium in cultured rat renal arterial smooth muscle cells. Clin Exp Pharmacol Physiol. 1996;23(6-7):503–507. doi:10.1111/j.1440-1681.1996.tb02769.x

537 Pellegatti P, Raffaghello L, Bianchi G, Piccardi F, Pistoia V, Di Virgilio F (2008) Increased Level of Extracellular ATP at Tumor Sites: In Vivo Imaging with Plasma Membrane Luciferase. PLoS ONE 3(7): e2599. https://doi.org/10.1371/journal.pone.0002599

538 Shi Y, Pestka JJ. Mechanisms for suppression of interleukin-6 expression in peritoneal macrophages from docosahexaenoic acid-fed mice. J Nutr Biochem. 2009;20(5):358–368. doi:10.1016/j.jnutbio.2008.04.006

539 García-Escobar E, Rodríguez-Pacheco F, García-Serrano S, et al. Nutritional regulation of interleukin-6 release from adipocytes. Int J Obes (Lond). 2010;34(8):1328–1332. doi:10.1038/ijo.2010.70

540 Sandeep R. Varma, Thiyagarajan O. Sivaprakasam, Ilavarasu Arumugam, N. Dilip, M. Raghuraman, K.B. Pavan, Mohammed Rafiq, Rangesh Paramesh, In vitro anti-inflammatory and skin protective properties of Virgin coconut oil, Journal of Traditional and Complementary Medicine, Volume 9, Issue 1, 2019, Pages 5-14, ISSN 2225-4110, https://doi.org/10.1016/j.jtcme.2017.06.012

541 Ling PR, Malkan A, Le HD, Puder M, Bistrian BR. Arachidonic acid and docosahexaenoic acid supplemented to an essential fatty acid-deficient diet alters the response to endotoxin in rats. Metabolism. 2012;61(3):395–406. doi:10.1016/j.metabol.2011.07.017

542 Shen Y, Wan H, Zhu J, et al. Fish Oil and Olive Oil Supplementation in Late Pregnancy and Lactation Differentially Affect Oxidative Stress and Inflammation in Sows and Piglets. Lipids. 2015;50(7):647–658. doi:10.1007/s11745-015-4024-x

543 Li, H., Zhu, Y., Zhao, F. et al. Fish oil, lard and soybean oil differentially shape gut microbiota of middle-aged rats. Sci Rep 7, 826 (2017). https://doi.org/10.1038/s41598-017-00969-0

544 Vaisman, Nachum & Zaruk, Yahalomit & Shirazi, Idit & Kaysar, Nechemia & Barak, Vivian. (2005). The effect of fish oil supplementation on cytokine production in children. European cytokine network. 16. 194-8

545 Muldoon MF, Laderian B, Kuan DC, Sereika SM, Marsland AL, Manuck SB. Fish oil supplementation does not lower C-reactive protein or interleukin-6

levels in healthy adults. J Intern Med. 2016;279(1):98-109. doi:10.1111/joim.12442

546 Spickett, Corinne & Jerlich, A & Panasenko, O.M. & Arnhold, Jürgen & Pitt, Andrew & Stelmaszyńska, T & Schaur, Rudolf. (2000). The reactions of hypoclorous acid, the reactive oxygen species produced by myeloperoxidase, with lipids. Acta biochimica Polonica. 47. 889-99. 10.18388/abp.2000_3944

547 Thukkani AK, McHowat J, Hsu FF, Brennan ML, Hazen SL, Ford DA. Identification of alpha-chloro fatty aldehydes and unsaturated lysophosphatidylcholine molecular species in human atherosclerotic lesions. Circulation. 2003;108(25):3128–3133. doi:10.1161/01.CIR.0000104564.01539.6A

548 Yue L, Pang Z, Li H, Yang T, Guo L, Liu L, et al. (2018) CXCL4 contributes to host defense against acute Pseudomonas aeruginosa lung infection. PLoS ONE 13(10): e0205521. https://doi.org/10.1371/journal.pone.0205521

549 Tidy, L. (1928) The haemorrhagic diathesis. Proceedings of the Royal Society of Medicine, 21, 1033–1052

550 Zhang, Xin & Liu, Yu & Gao, Yaping & Dong, Jie & Mu, Chunhua & Lu, Qiang & Shao, Ningsheng & Yang, Guang. (2011). Inhibiting platelets aggregation could aggravate the acute infection caused by Staphylococcus aureus. Platelets. 22. 228-36. 10.3109/09537104.2010.543962

551 Adam R. Berliner, Derek M. Fine, There's something fishy about this bleeding, NDT Plus, Volume 4, Issue 4, August 2011, Pages 270–272, https://doi.org/10.1093/ndtplus/sfr046

552 August Bagge, Ulf Schött & Thomas Kander (2018) High-dose omega-3 fatty acids have no effect on platelet aggregation or coagulation measured with static and flow-based aggregation instruments and Sonoclot; an observational study in healthy volunteers, Scandinavian Journal of Clinical and Laboratory Investigation, 78:7-8, 539-545, DOI: 10.1080/00365513.2018.1516477

553 Roy K, Mandloi S, Chakrabarti S, Roy S. Cholesterol Corrects Altered Conformation of MHC-II Protein in Leishmania donovani Infected Macrophages: Implication in Therapy. PLoS Negl Trop Dis. 2016;10(5):e0004710. Published 2016 May 23. doi:10.1371/journal.pntd.0004710

554 Netea MG, Joosten LA, Keuter M, et al. Circulating lipoproteins are a crucial component of host defense against invasive Salmonella typhimurium infection. PLoS One. 2009;4(1):e4237. doi:10.1371/journal.pone.0004237

555 Pajkrt D, Doran JE, Koster F, et al. Antiinflammatory effects of reconstituted high-density lipoprotein during human endotoxemia. J Exp Med. 1996;184(5):1601–1608. doi:10.1084/jem.184.5.1601

556 Harris HW, Grunfeld C, Feingold KR, Rapp JH. Human very low density lipoproteins and chylomicrons can protect against endotoxin-induced death in mice. J Clin Invest. 1990;86(3):696–702. doi:10.1172/JCI114765

557 Huemer HP, Menzel HJ, Potratz D, et al. Herpes simplex virus binds to human serum lipoprotein. Intervirology. 1988;29(2):68–76. doi:10.1159/000150031

558 558 Albert AD, Boesze-Battaglia K, Paw Z, Watts A, Epand RM. Effect of cholesterol on rhodopsin stability in disk membranes. Biochim Biophys Acta. 1996;1297(1):77–82. doi:10.1016/0167-4838(96)00102-1

559 Parasassi T, Giusti AM, Raimondi M, Ravagnan G, Sapora O, Gratton E. Cholesterol protects the phospholipid bilayer from oxidative damage. Free Radic Biol Med. 1995;19(4):511–516. doi:10.1016/0891-5849(95)00038-y

560 Samuni AM, Lipman A, Barenholz Y. Damage to liposomal lipids: protection by antioxidants and cholesterol-mediated dehydration. Chem Phys Lipids. 2000;105(2):121–134. doi:10.1016/s0009-3084(99)00136-x

561 Pfohl M, Schreiber I, Liebich HM, Häring HU, Hoffmeister HM. Upregulation of cholesterol synthesis after acute myocardial infarction--is cholesterol a positive acute phase reactant?. Atherosclerosis. 1999;142(2):389–393. doi:10.1016/s0021-9150(98)00242-1

562 Cannon CP, Braunwald E, McCabe CH, et al. Intensive versus moderate lipid lowering with statins after acute coronary syndromes [published correction appears in N Engl J Med. 2006 Feb 16;354(7):778]. N Engl J Med. 2004;350(15):1495-1504. doi:10.1056/NEJMoa040583

563 Vaughan CJ, Murphy MB, Buckley BM. Statins do more than just lower cholesterol [published correction appears in Lancet 1997 Jan 18;349(9046):214]. Lancet. 1996;348(9034):1079-1082. doi:10.1016/S0140-6736(96)05190-2

564 Weis M, Pehlivanli S, Meiser BM, von Scheidt W. Simvastatin treatment is associated with improvement in coronary endothelial function and decreased cytokine activation in patients after heart transplantation. J Am Coll Cardiol. 2001;38(3):814-818. doi:10.1016/s0735-1097(01)01430-9

565 Hecht HS, Harman SM. Relation of aggressiveness of lipid-lowering treatment to changes in calcified plaque burden by electron beam tomography. Am J Cardiol. 2003;92(3):334–336. doi:10.1016/s0002-9149(03)00642-8

566 Ando H, Takamura T, Ota T, Nagai Y, Kobayashi K. Cerivastatin improves survival of mice with lipopolysaccharide-induced sepsis. J Pharmacol Exp Ther. 2000;294(3):1043-1046

567 Bouitbir J, Charles AL, Rasseneur L, et al. Atorvastatin treatment reduces exercise capacities in rats: involvement of mitochondrial impairments and oxidative stress. J Appl Physiol (1985). 2011;111(5):1477-1483. doi:10.1152/japplphysiol.00107.2011

568 Ziad A. Massy, Carlos Guijarro, Statins: effects beyond cholesterol lowering, Nephrology Dialysis Transplantation, Volume 16, Issue 9, September 2001, Pages 1738–1741, https://doi.org/10.1093/ndt/16.9.1738

569 Bietz A, Zhu H, Xue M and Xu C (2017) Cholesterol Metabolism in T Cells. Front. Immunol. 8:1664. doi: 10.3389/fimmu.2017.01664

570 STROM A, JENSEN RA. Mortality from circulatory diseases in Norway 1940-1945. Lancet. 1951;1(6647):126–129. doi:10.1016/s0140-6736(51)91210-x

571 Bang HO, Dyerberg J, Nielsen AB. Plasma lipid and lipoprotein pattern in Greenlandic West-coast Eskimos. Lancet. 1971;1(7710):1143–1145. doi:10.1016/s0140-6736(71)91658-8

572 Dyerberg J, Bang HO, Stoffersen E, Moncada S, Vane JR. Eicosapentaenoic acid and prevention of thrombosis and atherosclerosis?. Lancet. 1978;2(8081):117-119. doi:10.1016/s0140-6736(78)91505-2

573 Kromhout D, Bosschieter EB, de Lezenne Coulander C. The inverse relation between fish consumption and 20-year mortality from coronary heart disease. N Engl J Med. 1985;312(19):1205-1209. doi:10.1056/NEJM198505093121901

574 'De cardiologie heeft ons ingehaald' 25 JAAR STUDIE NAAR VETZUREN UIT VIS. VOEDING EN GEZONDHEID. Wageningen world. "authors translation"

575 Risk and Prevention Study Collaborative Group, Roncaglioni MC, Tombesi M, et al. n-3 fatty acids in patients with multiple cardiovascular risk factors [published correction appears in N Engl J Med. 2013 May 30;368(22):2146]. N Engl J Med. 2013;368(19):1800-1808. doi:10.1056/NEJMoa1205409

576 Burr ML, Ashfield-Watt PA, Dunstan FD, et al. Lack of benefit of dietary advice to men with angina: results of a controlled trial. Eur J Clin Nutr. 2003;57(2):193–200. doi:10.1038/sj.ejcn.1601539

577 Kromhout D, Giltay EJ, Geleijnse JM; Alpha Omega Trial Group. n-3 fatty acids and cardiovascular events after myocardial infarction. N Engl J Med. 2010;363(21):2015–2026. doi:10.1056/NEJMoa1003603

578 Hoogeveen EK, Geleijnse JM, Kromhout D, et al. No effect of n-3 fatty acids supplementation on NT-proBNP after myocardial infarction: the Alpha Omega Trial. Eur J Prev Cardiol. 2015;22(5):648-655. doi:10.1177/2047487314536694

579 Hoogeveen, Ellen & Geleijnse, Johanna & Kromhout, Daan & Giltay, Erik. (2013). No effect of n-3 fatty acids on high-sensitivity C-reactive protein after myocardial infarction: The Alpha Omega Trial. European journal of preventive cardiology. 21. 10.1177/2047487313494295

580 Galan, Pilar & Kesse-Guyot, Emmanuelle & Czernichow, Sebastien & Briançon, Serge & Blacher, Jacques & Hercberg, Serge. (2010). Effects of B vitamins and omega 3 fatty acids on cardiovascular diseases: a randomised placebo controlled trialSU.FOL.OM3 Collaborative GroupBMJ2010341c627310.1136/bmj.c6273299304521115589. BMJ (Clinical research ed.). 341. c6273. 10.1136/bmj.c6273.

581 Claudia M Oomen, Marga C Ocké, Edith JM Feskens, Frans J Kok, Daan Kromhout, α-Linolenic acid intake is not beneficially associated with 10-y risk of coronary artery disease incidence: the Zutphen Elderly Study, The American Journal of Clinical Nutrition, Volume 74, Issue 4, October 2001, Pages 457–463, https://doi.org/10.1093/ajcn/74.4.457

582 Amiano P, Machón M, Dorronsoro M, et al. Intake of total omega-3 fatty acids, eicosapentaenoic acid and docosahexaenoic acid and risk of coronary heart disease in the Spanish EPIC cohort study. Nutr Metab Cardiovasc Dis. 2014;24(3):321–327. doi:10.1016/j.numecd.2013.08.011

583 Ascherio A, Rimm EB, Stampfer MJ, Giovannucci EL, Willett WC. Dietary intake of marine n-3 fatty acids, fish intake, and the risk of coronary disease among men. N Engl J Med. 1995;332(15):977–982. doi:10.1056/NEJM199504133321501

584 Rauch B, Schiele R, Schneider S, Diller F, Victor N, Gohlke H, Gottwik M, Steinbeck G, Del Castillo U, Sack R, Worth H, Katus H, Spitzer W, Sabin G, Senges J, OMEGA Study Group. OMEGA, a randomized, placebo-controlled trial to test the effect of highly purified omega-3 fatty acids on top of modern guideline-adjusted therapy after myocardial infarction. Circulation. 2010 Nov;122(21) 2152-2159. doi:10.1161/circulationaha.110.948562. PMID: 21060071

585 Angerer P, Kothny W, Störk S, von Schacky C. Effect of dietary supplementation with omega-3 fatty acids on progression of atherosclerosis

in carotid arteries. Cardiovasc Res. 2002;54(1):183–190. doi:10.1016/s0008-6363(02)00229-8

586 Raitt MH, Connor WE, Morris C, et al. Fish oil supplementation and risk of ventricular tachycardia and ventricular fibrillation in patients with implantable defibrillators: a randomized controlled trial. JAMA. 2005;293(23):2884–2891. doi:10.1001/jama.293.23.2884

587 Guallar E, Hennekens CH, Sacks FM, Willett WC, Stampfer MJ. A prospective study of plasma fish oil levels and incidence of myocardial infarction in U.S. male physicians. J Am Coll Cardiol. 1995;25(2):387–394. doi:10.1016/0735-1097(94)00370-6

588 Poppitt SD, Howe CA, Lithander FE, et al. Effects of moderate-dose omega-3 fish oil on cardiovascular risk factors and mood after ischemic stroke: a randomized, controlled trial. Stroke. 2009;40(11):3485–3492. doi:10.1161/STROKEAHA.109.555136

589 Daneshmand R, Kurl S, Tuomainen TP, Virtanen JK. Associations of serum n-3 and n-6 PUFA and hair mercury with the risk of incident stroke in men: the Kuopio Ischaemic Heart Disease Risk Factor Study (KIHD). Br J Nutr. 2016;115(10):1851–1859. doi:10.1017/S0007114516000982

590 Billman GE, Carnes CA, Adamson PB, Vanoli E, Schwartz PJ. Dietary omega-3 fatty acids and susceptibility to ventricular fibrillation: lack of protection and a proarrhythmic effect [published correction appears in Circ Arrhythm Electrophysiol. 2012 Aug 1;5(4):e89]. Circ Arrhythm Electrophysiol. 2012;5(3):553–560. doi:10.1161/CIRCEP.111.966739

591 Carbone A, Psaltis PJ, Nelson AJ, et al. Dietary omega-3 supplementation exacerbates left ventricular dysfunction in an ovine model of anthracycline-induced cardiotoxicity. J Card Fail. 2012;18(6):502–511. doi:10.1016/j.cardfail.2012.03.005

592 Kirkeby K, Ingvaldsen P, Bjerkedal I. Fatty acid composition of serum lipids in men with myocardial infarction. Acta Med Scand. 1972;192(6):513–519. doi:10.1111/j.0954-6820.1972.tb04857.x

593 Galvao TF, Brown BH, Hecker PA, et al. High intake of saturated fat, but not polyunsaturated fat, improves survival in heart failure despite persistent mitochondrial defects. Cardiovasc Res. 2012;93(1):24–32. doi:10.1093/cvr/cvr258

594 Galvao TF, Khairallah RJ, Dabkowski ER, et al. Marine n3 polyunsaturated fatty acids enhance resistance to mitochondrial permeability transition in

heart failure but do not improve survival. Am J Physiol Heart Circ Physiol. 2013;304(1):H12–H21. doi:10.1152/ajpheart.00657.2012

595 Brouwer IA, Zock PL, Camm AJ, et al. Effect of fish oil on ventricular tachyarrhythmia and death in patients with implantable cardioverter defibrillators: the Study on Omega-3 Fatty Acids and Ventricular Arrhythmia (SOFA) randomized trial. JAMA. 2006;295(22):2613–2619. doi:10.1001/jama.295.22.2613

596 Bianconi L, Calò L, Mennuni M, et al. n-3 polyunsaturated fatty acids for the prevention of arrhythmia recurrence after electrical cardioversion of chronic persistent atrial fibrillation: a randomized, double-blind, multicentre study. Europace. 2011;13(2):174–181. doi:10.1093/europace/euq386

597 Brouwer, Ingeborg & Raitt, Merritt & Dullemeijer, Carla & Kraemer, Dale & Zock, Peter & Morris, Cynthia & Katan, Martijn & Connor, William & Camm, John & Schouten, Evert & Mcanulty, John. (2009). Effect of fish oil on ventricular tachyarrhythmia in three studies in patients with implantable cardioverter defibrillators. European heart journal. 30. 820-6. 10.1093/eurheartj/ehp003

598 Moreno C, Macías A, Prieto A, de la Cruz A, González T, Valenzuela C. Effects of n-3 Polyunsaturated Fatty Acids on Cardiac Ion Channels. Front Physiol. 2012;3:245. Published 2012 Jul 9. doi:10.3389/fphys.2012.00245

599 Xu X, Jiang M, Wang Y, Smith T, Baumgarten CM, Wood MA, et al. (2010) Long-Term Fish Oil Supplementation Induces Cardiac Electrical Remodeling by Changing Channel Protein Expression in the Rabbit Model. PLoS ONE 5(4): e10140. https://doi.org/10.1371/journal.pone.0010140

600 Htun P, Nee J, Ploeckinger U, Eder K, Geisler T, Gawaz M, et al. (2015) Fish-Free Diet in Patients with Phenylketonuria Is Not Associated with Early Atherosclerotic Changes and Enhanced Platelet Activation. PLoS ONE 10(8): e0135930. https://doi.org/10.1371/journal.pone.0135930

601 Mabile L, Salvayre R, Bonnafé MJ, Nègre-Salvayre A. Oxidizability and subsequent cytotoxicity of chylomicrons to monocytic U937 and endothelial cells are dependent on dietary fatty acid composition. Free Radic Biol Med. 1995 Nov;19(5) 599-607. doi:10.1016/0891-5849(95)00070-e. PMID: 8529919

602 Ringseis, R. and Eder, K. (2003), Effects of dietary fish oil and oxidized cholesterol on the concentration of 7β-hydroxycholesterol in liver, plasma, low density lipoproteins and erythrocytes of rats at various vitamin E supply. Eur. J. Lipid Sci. Technol., 105: 121-129. doi:10.1002/ejlt.200390027

603 Suzukawa M, Abbey M, Howe PR, Nestel PJ. Effects of fish oil fatty acids on low density lipoprotein size, oxidizability, and uptake by macrophages. J Lipid Res. 1995;36(3):473–484

604 Nishi K, Itabe H, Uno M, et al. Oxidized LDL in carotid plaques and plasma associates with plaque instability. Arterioscler Thromb Vasc Biol. 2002;22(10):1649–1654. doi:10.1161/01.atv.0000033829.14012.18

605 Colas R, Pruneta-Deloche V, Guichardant M, et al. Increased lipid peroxidation in LDL from type-2 diabetic patients. Lipids. 2010;45(8):723–731. doi:10.1007/s11745-010-3453-9

606 Pedersen H, Petersen M, Major-Pedersen A, et al. Influence of fish oil supplementation on in vivo and in vitro oxidation resistance of low-density lipoprotein in type 2 diabetes. Eur J Clin Nutr. 2003;57(5):713–720. doi:10.1038/sj.ejcn.1601602

607 Frankel EN, Parks EJ, Xu R, Schneeman BO, Davis PA, German JB. Effect of n-3 fatty acid-rich fish oil supplementation on the oxidation of low density lipoproteins. Lipids. 1994;29(4):233–236. doi:10.1007/bf02536326

608 Lussier-Cacan S, Dubreuil-Quidoz S, Roederer G, et al. Influence of probucol on enhanced LDL oxidation after fish oil treatment of hypertriglyceridemic patients. Arterioscler Thromb. 1993;13(12):1790–1797. doi:10.1161/01.atv.13.12.1790

609 Korpela R, Seppo L, Laakso J, et al. Dietary habits affect the susceptibility of low-density lipoprotein to oxidation. Eur J Clin Nutr. 1999;53(10):802–807. doi:10.1038/sj.ejcn.1600860

610 M-Shirazi M, Taleban FA, Abadi AR, Sabetkasaei M. Fish oil increases atherosclerosis and hepatic steatosis, although decreases serum cholesterol in Wistar rat. J Res Med Sci. 2011;16(5):583–590

611 Ritskes-Hoitinga J, Verschuren PM, Meijer GW, et al. The association of increasing dietary concentrations of fish oil with hepatotoxic effects and a higher degree of aorta atherosclerosis in the ad lib.-fed rabbit. Food Chem Toxicol. 1998;36(8):663–672. doi:10.1016/s0278-6915(98)00028-3

612 Verschuren PM, Houtsmuller UM, Zevenbergen JL. Evaluation of vitamin E requirement and food palatability in rabbits fed a purified diet with a high fish oil content. Lab Anim. 1990;24(2):164–171. doi:10.1258/002367790780890167

613 Nalbone G, Termine E, Léonardi J, et al. Effect of dietary salmon oil feeding on rat heart lipid status. J Nutr. 1988;118(7):809–817. doi:10.1093/jn/118.7.809

614 Lemieux H, Bulteau AL, Friguet B, Tardif JC, Blier PU. Dietary fatty acids and oxidative stress in the heart mitochondria. Mitochondrion. 2011;11(1):97–103. doi:10.1016/j.mito.2010.07.014

615 Mohsen Meydani et al. Effect of Long-Term Fish Oil Supplementation on Vitamin E Status and Lipid Peroxidation in Women. The Journal of Nutrition (1991) 121 (4): 484-491. By permission of Oxford University Press on behalf of The American Institute of Nutrition. Available at: https://academic.oup.com/jn/article/121/4/484/4754632?searchresult=1

616 Bietz A, Zhu H, Xue M and Xu C (2017) Cholesterol Metabolism in T Cells. Front. Immunol. 8:1664. doi: 10.3389/fimmu.2017.01664

617 Jeong S-M, Choi S, Kim K, Kim S-M, Lee G, Son JS, et al. (2018) Association of change in total cholesterol level with mortality: A population-based study. PLoS ONE 13(4): e0196030. https://doi.org/10.1371/journal.pone.0196030

618 Hoenselaar R. Saturated fat and cardiovascular disease: the discrepancy between the scientific literature and dietary advice. Nutrition. 2012;28(2):118-123. doi:10.1016/j.nut.2011.08.017

619 National Research Council (US) Committee on Diet, Nutrition, and Cancer. Diet, Nutrition, and Cancer. Washington (DC): National Academies Press (US); 1982

620 Bowe B, Xie Y, Xian H, Balasubramanian S, Zayed MA, Al-Aly Z. High Density Lipoprotein Cholesterol and the Risk of All-Cause Mortality among U.S. Veterans. Clin J Am Soc Nephrol. 2016;11(10):1784–1793. doi:10.2215/CJN.00730116

621 Ravnskov U, Diamond DM, Hama R, et al. Lack of an association or an inverse association between low-density-lipoprotein cholesterol and mortality in the elderly: a systematic review. BMJ Open. 2016;6(6):e010401. Published 2016 Jun 12. doi:10.1136/bmjopen-2015-010401

622 Zanoni P, Khetarpal SA, Larach DB, et al. Rare variant in scavenger receptor BI raises HDL cholesterol and increases risk of coronary heart disease. Science. 2016;351(6278):1166–1171. doi:10.1126/science.aad3517

623 Zanoni P, Khetarpal SA, Larach DB, et al. Rare variant in scavenger receptor BI raises HDL cholesterol and increases risk of coronary heart disease. Science. 2016;351(6278):1166–1171. doi:10.1126/science.aad3517

624 Horwich TB, Hamilton MA, Maclellan WR, Fonarow GC. Low serum total cholesterol is associated with marked increase in mortality in advanced heart failure. J Card Fail. 2002;8(4):216–224. doi:10.1054/jcaf.2002.0804216

625 Brescianini S, Maggi S, Farchi G, et al. Low total cholesterol and increased risk of dying: are low levels clinical warning signs in the elderly? Results from the Italian Longitudinal Study on Aging. J Am Geriatr Soc. 2003;51(7):991–996. doi:10.1046/j.1365-2389.2003.51313.x

626 West R, Beeri MS, Schmeidler J, et al. Better memory functioning associated with higher total and low-density lipoprotein cholesterol levels in very elderly subjects without the apolipoprotein e4 allele. Am J Geriatr Psychiatry. 2008;16(9):781–785. doi:10.1097/JGP.0b013e3181812790

627 Cabrera, Marcos & Andrade, Selma & Dip, Renata. (2012). Lipids and All-Cause Mortality among Older Adults: A 12-Year Follow-Up Study. TheScientificWorldJournal. 2012. 930139. 10.1100/2012/930139

628 Tuikkala P, Hartikainen S, Korhonen MJ, et al. Serum total cholesterol levels and all-cause mortality in a home-dwelling elderly population: a six-year follow-up. Scand J Prim Health Care. 2010;28(2):121–127. doi:10.3109/02813432.2010.487371

629 Iseki K, Yamazato M, Tozawa M, Takishita S. Hypocholesterolemia is a significant predictor of death in a cohort of chronic hemodialysis patients. Kidney Int. 2002;61(5):1887–1893. doi:10.1046/j.1523-1755.2002.00324.x

630 Saito N, Sairenchi T, Irie F, et al. Low serum LDL cholesterol levels are associated with elevated mortality from liver cancer in Japan: the Ibaraki Prefectural health study. Tohoku J Exp Med. 2013;229(3):203–211. doi:10.1620/tjem.229.203

631 Akerblom JL, Costa R, Luchsinger JA, et al. Relation of plasma lipids to all-cause mortality in Caucasian, African-American and Hispanic elders. Age Ageing. 2008;37(2):207–213. doi:10.1093/ageing/afn017

632 Liu CY, Chou YC, Lin SH, et al. Serum lipid profiles are associated with semen quality. Asian J Androl. 2017;19(6):633–638. doi:10.4103/1008-682X.195240

633 Spinarova L, Spinar J, Vitovec J, et al. Gender differences in total cholesterol levels in patients with acute heart failure and its importance for short and long time prognosis. Biomed Pap Med Fac Univ Palacky Olomouc Czech Repub. 2012;156(1):21–28. doi:10.5507/bp.2012.015

634 Afshinnia F, Chacko S, Zahedi T. Association of lower serum cholesterol levels with higher risk of osteoporosis in type 2 diabetes. Endocr Pract. 2007;13(6):620–628. doi:10.4158/EP.13.6.620

635 Wang X, Dong Y, Qi X, Huang C, Hou L. Cholesterol levels and risk of hemorrhagic stroke: a systematic review and meta-analysis. Stroke. 2013;44(7):1833–1839. doi:10.1161/STROKEAHA.113.001326

636 Andreo U, Elkind J, Blachford C, Cederbaum AI, Fisher EA. Role of superoxide radical anion in the mechanism of apoB100 degradation induced by DHA in hepatic cells. FASEB J. 2011;25(10):3554-3560. doi:10.1096/fj.11-182725

637 Goldberg IJ, Huang LS, Huggins LA, et al. Thyroid hormone reduces cholesterol via a non-LDL receptor-mediated pathway. Endocrinology. 2012;153(11):5143-5149. doi:10.1210/en.2012-1572

638 Anitschkow N (1913) Über die Veränderungen der Kaninchenaorta bei experimenteller Cholesterinsteatose. Beitr Pathol Anat 56: 379–404

639 Clarkson S, Newburgh LH. THE RELATION BETWEEN ATHEROSCLEROSIS AND INGESTED CHOLESTEROL IN THE RABBIT. J Exp Med. 1926;43(5):595-612. doi:10.1084/jem.43.5.595

640 Cook, R. P., McCullagh, G. P., (1939), A COMPARATIVE STUDY OF CHOLESTEROL METABOLISM AND ITS RELATION TO FATTY INFILTRATION, WITH PARTICULAR REFERENCE TO EXPERIMENTAL CHOLESTEROL ATHEROMA. Experimental Physiology, 29 doi: 10.1113/expphysiol.1939.sp000809

641 Turner KB. STUDIES ON THE PREVENTION OF CHOLESTEROL ATHEROSCLEROSIS IN RABBITS : I. THE EFFECTS OF WHOLE THYROID AND OF POTASSIUM IODIDE. J Exp Med. 1933;58(1):115-125. doi:10.1084/jem.58.1.115

642 McLETCHIE NG. The pathogenesis of atheroma. Am J Pathol. 1952;28(3):413-435

643 OLIVER MF, BOYD GS. Influence of reduction of serum lipids on prognosis of coronary heart-disease. A five-year study using oestrogen. Lancet. 1961;2(7201):499-505. doi:10.1016/s0140-6736(61)92951-8

644 [The influence of nutrition and way of life on physical condition, serum cholesterol content and incidence of atherosclerosis and coronary thrombosis in Trappist and Benedictine monks]. GROEN JJ, TJIONG BK, KOSTER M, VERDONCK G, PIERLOOT R, WILLEBRANDS AF. Ned Tijdschr Geneeskd. 1961 Feb 4;105:222-33. Dutch

645 PAGE IH, STARE FJ, CORCORAN AC, POLLACK H, WILKINSON CF Jr. Atherosclerosis and the fat content of the diet. Circulation. 1957;16(2):163-178. doi:10.1161/01.cir.16.2.163

646 Maurice Bruger, M.D., J. A. Rosenkrantz, M.D., Arteriosclerosis and Hypothyroidism: Observations on Their Possible Interrelationship, The

Journal of Clinical Endocrinology & Metabolism, Volume 2, Issue 3, 1 March 1942, Pages 176–180, https://doi.org/10.1210/jcem-2-3-176

647 STEINER A, KENDALL FE. Atherosclerosis and arteriosclerosis in dogs following ingestion of cholesterol and thiouracil. Arch Pathol (Chic). 1946;42(4):433–444

648 Spinar J, Ludka O, Senkyríková M, Vítovec J, Spinarová L, Dusek L. Hladiny cholesterolu v závislosti na veku [Cholesterol levels according to age]. Vnitr Lek. 2009;55(9):724–729

649 Cholesterol.David Kritchevsky. New York, John Wiley & Sons, Inc., 1958. pp.291, $9.75, Clinical Chemistry, Volume 5, Issue 6, 1 December 1959, Page 635, https://doi.org/10.1093/clinchem/5.6.635b

650 GLAVIND J, HARTMANN S, CLEMMESEN J, JESSEN KE, DAM H. Studies on the role of lipoperoxides in human pathology. II. The presence of peroxidized lipids in the atherosclerotic aorta. Acta Pathol Microbiol Scand. 1952;30(1):1–6. doi:10.1111/j.1699-0463.1952.tb00157.x

651 Werken aan scheikunde, 24 memoires van hen die de Nederlandse Chemie deze eeuw groot hebben gemaakt. Uitgegeven door Delftse Universitaire Pers in 1993. (Copyright 1993 by Delft University Pers). Own translation

652 Böttcher C, J, F: Chemical Factors in Atherogenesis. Pathobiology 1967;30:619-628. doi: 10.1159/000161702

653 NATUURKUNDIGE VOORDRACHTEN 1960 – 1961. NIEUWE REEK S No . 39 VOORDRACHTEN GEHOUDEN VOOR DE KONINKLIJKE MAATSCHAPPIJ DILIGENTIA. TE S-GRAVENHAGE OPGERICHT 1793 BESCHERMVROUW H.M, DE KONINGIN

654 The Patient Has the Floor* ALISTAIR COOKE. Address given before the Annual Convocation of the Mayo Graduate School of Medicine, Rochester, Minnesota, on May 28, 1965. The Mayo Clinic Proceedings 41: 103-113 (Feb.), 1966.Chief United States Correspondent, The Guardian, ISBN 1555042147 (ISBN13: 9781555042141)

655 Council on foodsand nutritions (1958) J.Amer.med, Ass. 167, 863

656 Bondjers G, Björkerud S. Cholesterol accumulation and content in regions with defined endothelial integrity in the normal rabbit aorta. Atherosclerosis. 1973;17(1):71-83. doi:10.1016/0021-9150(73)90136-6

657 Iwakami M. Peroxides as a factor of atherosclerosis. Nagoya J Med Sci. 1965;28(1):50–66

658 ARTHUR F. WHEREAT TI - Oxygen Consumption of Normal and Atherosclerotic Intima PT - Journal Article DP - 1961 TA - Circulation

Research PG - 571-575 VI - 9 IP - 3 AID - 10.1161/01.RES.9.3.571 [doi] 4099 - https://www.ahajournals.org/doi/abs/10.1161/01.RES.9.3.571 4100 -

659 Stringer MD, Görög PG, Freeman A, Kakkar VV. Lipid peroxides and atherosclerosis. BMJ. 1989;298(6669):281-284. doi:10.1136/bmj.298.6669.281

660 Signorini C, De Felice C, Durand T, et al. Isoprostanes and 4-hydroxy-2-nonenal: markers or mediators of disease? Focus on Rett syndrome as a model of autism spectrum disorder. Oxid Med Cell Longev. 2013;2013:343824. doi:10.1155/2013/343824

661 ROSE GA, THOMSON WB, WILLIAMS RT. CORN OIL IN TREATMENT OF ISCHAEMIC HEART DISEASE. Br Med J. 1965;1(5449):1531-1533. doi:10.1136/bmj.1.5449.1531

662 Ramsden CE, Zamora D, Leelarthaepin B, et al. Use of dietary linoleic acid for secondary prevention of coronary heart disease and death: evaluation of recovered data from the Sydney Diet Heart Study and updated meta-analysis. BMJ 2013;346:e8707 10.1136/bmj.e8707

663 Ramsden CE, Zamaora D, Majchrzak-Hong S, et al. Re-evaluation of the traditional diet-heart hypothesis: analysis of recovered data from Minnesota Coronary Experiment (1968-73). BMJ 2016;352:i1246

664 MOHAMED A. ANTAR, M.B.B.CH., M.S., MARGARET A. OHLSON, PH.D., ROBERT E. HODGES, M.D., Changes in Retail Market Food Supplies in the United States in the Last Seventy Years in Relation to the Incidence of Coronary Heart Disease, with Special Reference to Dietary Carbohydrates and Essential Fatty Acids, The American Journal of Clinical Nutrition, Volume 14, Issue 3, March 1964, Pages 169–178, https://doi.org/10.1093/ajcn/14.3.169

665 J. Thiery, D. Seidel, Fish oil feeding results in an enhancement of cholesterol-induced atherosclerosis in rabbits, Atherosclerosis, Volume 63, Issue 1, 1987, Pages 53-56, ISSN 0021-9150, https://doi.org/10.1016/0021-9150(87)90081-5. (http://www.sciencedirect.com/science/article/pii/0021915087900815)

666 Chen Y-W, Li C-H, Yang C-D, Liu C-H, Chen C-H, Sheu J-J, et al. (2017) Low cholesterol level associated with severity and outcome of spontaneous intracerebral hemorrhage: Results from Taiwan Stroke Registry. PLoS ONE 12(4): e0171379. https://doi.org/10.1371/journal.pone.0171379

667 Suominen-Taipale AL, Partonen T, Turunen AW, Männistö S, Jula A, Verkasalo PK (2010) Fish Consumption and Omega-3 Polyunsaturated Fatty Acids in Relation to Depressive Episodes: A Cross-Sectional Analysis. PLoS ONE 5(5): e10530. https://doi.org/10.1371/journal.pone.0010530

668 Assies J, Pouwer F, Lok A, Mocking RJT, Bockting CLH, Visser I, et al. (2010) Plasma and Erythrocyte Fatty Acid Patterns in Patients with Recurrent Depression: A Matched Case-Control Study. PLoS ONE 5(5): e10635. https://doi.org/10.1371/journal.pone.0010635

669 Pottala JV, Yaffe K, Robinson JG, Espeland MA, Wallace R, Harris WS. Higher RBC EPA + DHA corresponds with larger total brain and hippocampal volumes: WHIMS-MRI study. Neurology. 2014;82(5):435-442. doi:10.1212/WNL.0000000000000080

670 Abbott, Sarah & Jenner, Andrew & Spiro, Adena & Batterham, Marijka & Halliday, Glenda & Garner, Brett. (2015). Fatty Acid Composition of the Anterior Cingulate Cortex Indicates a High Susceptibility to Lipid Peroxidation in Parkinson's Disease. Journal of Parkinson's disease. 5. 10.3233/JPD-140479

671 Bate, C., Tayebi, M., Diomede, L. et al. Docosahexaenoic and eicosapentaenoic acids increase prion formation in neuronal cells . BMC Biol 6, 39 (2008). https://doi.org/10.1186/1741-7007-6-39

672 Bate C, Marshall V, Colombo L, Diomede L, Salmona M, Williams A. Docosahexaenoic and eicosapentaenoic acids increase neuronal death in response to HuPrP82-146 and Abeta 1-42. Neuropharmacology. 2008;54(6):934-943. doi:10.1016/j.neuropharm.2008.02.003

673 Braak E, Sandmann-Keil D, Rüb U, et al. alpha-synuclein immunopositive Parkinson's disease-related inclusion bodies in lower brain stem nuclei. Acta Neuropathol. 2001;101(3):195-201. doi:10.1007/s004010000247

674 Brummel BE, Braun AR, Sachs JN. Polyunsaturated chains in asymmetric lipids disorder raft mixtures and preferentially associate with α-Synuclein. Biochim Biophys Acta Biomembr. 2017;1859(4):529-536. doi:10.1016/j.bbamem.2016.10.006

675 De Franceschi G, Frare E, Pivato M, et al. Structural and morphological characterization of aggregated species of α-synuclein induced by docosahexaenoic acid. J Biol Chem. 2011;286(25):22262-22274. doi:10.1074/jbc.M110.202937

676 Broersen K, van den Brink D, Fraser G, Goedert M, Davletov B. Alpha-synuclein adopts an alpha-helical conformation in the presence of polyunsaturated fatty acids to hinder micelle formation. Biochemistry. 2006;45(51):15610-15616. doi:10.1021/bi061743l

677 De Franceschi G, Fecchio C, Sharon R, et al. α-Synuclein structural features inhibit harmful polyunsaturated fatty acid oxidation, suggesting roles in

neuroprotection. J Biol Chem. 2017;292(17):6927-6937. doi:10.1074/jbc. M116.765149

678 Amtul Z, Keet M, Wang L, Merrifield P, Westaway D, Rozmahel RF (2011) DHA Supplemented in Peptamen Diet Offers No Advantage in Pathways to Amyloidosis: Is It Time to Evaluate Composite Lipid Diet? PLoS ONE 6(9): e24094. https://doi.org/10.1371/journal.pone.0024094

679 Hsu YM, Yin MC. EPA or DHA enhanced oxidative stress and aging protein expression in brain of d-galactose treated mice. Biomedicine (Taipei). 2016;6(3):17. doi:10.7603/s40681-016-0017-1

680 Hillered L, Chan PH. Brain mitochondrial swelling induced by arachidonic acid and other long chain free fatty acids. J Neurosci Res. 1989;24(2):247-250. doi:10.1002/jnr.490240216

681 Calingasan NY, Uchida K, Gibson GE. Protein-bound acrolein: a novel marker of oxidative stress in Alzheimer's disease. Journal of Neurochemistry. 1999 Feb;72(2):751-756. DOI: 10.1046/j.1471-4159.1999.0720751.x

682 Miller, D., Leong, K. C., Knobl, G. M., & Gruger, E. (1964). Exudative Diathesis and Muscular Dystrophy Induced in the Chick by Esters of Polyunsaturated Fatty Acids. Proceedings of the Society for Experimental Biology and Medicine, 116(4), 1147–1151. https://doi.org/10.3181/00379727-116-29476

683 Pascoe MC, Howells DW, Crewther DP, Constantinou N, Carey LM, Rewell SS, Turchini GM, Kaur G and Crewther SG (2014) Fish oil diet associated with acute reperfusion related hemorrhage, and with reduced stroke-related sickness behaviors and motor impairment. Front. Neurol. 5:14. doi: 10.3389/fneur.2014.00014

684 Pascoe MC, Howells DW, Crewther DP, Constantinou N, Carey LM, Rewell SS, Turchini GM, Kaur G and Crewther SG (2014) Fish oil diet associated with acute reperfusion related hemorrhage, and with reduced stroke-related sickness behaviors and motor impairment. Front. Neurol. 5:14. doi: 10.3389/fneur.2014.00014

685 Long, E.K., Murphy, T.C., Leiphon, L.J., Watt, J., Morrow, J.D., Milne, G.L., Howard, J.R.H. and Picklo, M.J., Sr (2008), Trans-4-hydroxy-2-hexenal is a neurotoxic product of docosahexaenoic (22:6; n-3) acid oxidation. Journal of Neurochemistry, 105: 714-724. doi:10.1111/j.1471-4159.2007.05175.x

686 Markesbery WR, Kryscio RJ, Lovell MA, Morrow JD. Lipid peroxidation is an early event in the brain in amnestic mild cognitive impairment. Ann Neurol. 2005;58(5):730-735. doi:10.1002/ana.20629

687 Kristina Leuner, Susanne Hauptmann, Reham Abdel-Kader, Isabel Scherping, Uta Keil, Johanna B. Strosznajder, Anne Eckert, and Walter E. Müller.Antioxidants & Redox Signaling.Oct 2007.1659-1676.http://doi. org/10.1089/ars.2007.1763

688 Malis CD, Weber PC, Leaf A, Bonventre JV. Incorporation of marine lipids into mitochondrial membranes increases susceptibility to damage by calcium and reactive oxygen species: evidence for enhanced activation of phospholipase A2 in mitochondria enriched with n-3 fatty acids. Proc Natl Acad Sci U S A. 1990;87(22):8845-8849. doi:10.1073/pnas.87.22.8845

689 Snowden SG, Ebshiana AA, Hye A, et al. Association between fatty acid metabolism in the brain and Alzheimer disease neuropathology and cognitive performance: A nontargeted metabolomic study. PLoS Med. 2017;14(3):e1002266. Published 2017 Mar 21. doi:10.1371/journal. pmed.1002266

690 Yip PK, Pizzasegola C, Gladman S, Biggio ML, Marino M, Jayasinghe M, et al. (2013) The Omega-3 Fatty Acid Eicosapentaenoic Acid Accelerates Disease Progression in a Model of Amyotrophic Lateral Sclerosis. PLoS ONE 8(4): e61626. https://doi.org/10.1371/journal.pone.0061626

691 Bourre JM, Bonneil M, Dumont O, Piciotti M, Nalbone G, Lafont H. High dietary fish oil alters the brain polyunsaturated fatty acid composition. Biochim Biophys Acta. 1988;960(3):458-461. doi:10.1016/0005-2760(88)90055-0

692 Assies J, Pouwer F, Lok A, Mocking RJT, Bockting CLH, Visser I, et al. (2010) Plasma and Erythrocyte Fatty Acid Patterns in Patients with Recurrent Depression: A Matched Case-Control Study. PLoS ONE 5(5): e10635. https://doi.org/10.1371/journal.pone.0010635

693 Vaidya UV, Hegde VM, Bhave SA, Pandit AN. Vegetable oil fortified feeds in the nutrition of very low birthweight babies. Indian Pediatr. 1992;29(12):1519–1527

694 Philippe Grandjean, Kristian S Bjerve, Pál Weihe, Ulrike Steuerwald, Birthweight in a fishing community: significance of essential fatty acids and marine food contaminants, International Journal of Epidemiology, Volume 30, Issue 6, December 2001, Pages 1272–1278, https://doi. org/10.1093/ije/30.6.1272

695 Schock H, Zeleniuch-Jacquotte A, Lundin E, et al. Hormone concentrations throughout uncomplicated pregnancies: a longitudinal study. BMC

Pregnancy Childbirth. 2016;16(1):146. Published 2016 Jul 4. doi:10.1186/s12884-016-0937-5

696 Kauppila A, Kivelä A, Kontula K, Tuimala R. Serum progesterone, estradiol, and estriol before and during induced labor. Am J Obstet Gynecol. 1980;137(4):462-466. doi:10.1016/0002-9378(80)91129-1

697 Brenna JT, Varamini B, Jensen RG, Diersen-Schade DA, Boettcher JA, Arterburn LM. Docosahexaenoic and arachidonic acid concentrations in human breast milk worldwide. Am J Clin Nutr. 2007;85(6):1457-1464. doi:10.1093/ajcn/85.6.1457

698 Weisinger HS, Vingrys AJ, Abedin L, Sinclair AJ. Effect of diet on the rate of depletion of n-3 fatty acids in the retina of the guinea pig. J Lipid Res. 1998;39(6):1274-1279

699 Allen, J., & Wrieden, W. (1982). Influence of milk proteins on lipid oxidation in aqueous emulsion: I. Casein, whey protein and α-lactalbumin. Journal of Dairy Research, 49(2), 239-248. doi:10.1017/S0022029900022342

700 Genzel-Boroviczényy, O., Wahle, J. & Koletzko, B. Fatty acid composition of human milk during the 1st month after term and preterm delivery. Eur J Pediatr 156, 142–147 (1997). https://doi.org/10.1007/s004310050573

701 Liu CC, Carlson SE, Rhodes PG, Rao VS, Meydrech EF. Increase in plasma phospholipid docosahexaenoic and eicosapentaenoic acids as a reflection of their intake and mode of administration. Pediatr Res. 1987;22(3):292-296. doi:10.1203/00006450-198709000-00011

702 Santiago Burruchaga M, Ruiz Sanz JI, Pijoan Zubizarreta JI, Benito Fernández J, Sanjurjo Crespo P. Desarrollo intelectual en el segundo año de vida en niños sanos lactados de forma natural frente a los lactados artificialmente [Intellectual development in the second year of life in healthy breast-fed children compared with formula-fed children]. An Esp Pediatr. 2000;52(6):530-536.

703 Hibbeln JR, Davis JM, Steer C, et al. Maternal seafood consumption in pregnancy and neurodevelopmental outcomes in childhood (ALSPAC study): an observational cohort study. Lancet. 2007;369(9561):578-585. doi:10.1016/S0140-6736(07)60277-3

704 Carlson SE, Cooke RJ, Werkman SH, Tolley EA. First year growth of preterm infants fed standard compared to marine oil n-3 supplemented formula. Lipids. 1992;27(11):901-907. doi:10.1007/BF02535870

705 Goor, Saskia & Dijck-Brouwer, Janneke & Doornbos, Bennard & Erwich, Jan Jaap & Schaafsma, Anne & Muskiet, Frits & Hadders-Algra, Mijna.

(2009). Supplementation of DHA but not DHA with arachidonic acid during pregnancy and lactation influences general movement quality in 12-week-old term infants. The British journal of nutrition. 103. 235-42. 10.1017/S0007114509991528

706 de Jong C, Kikkert HK, Fidler V, Hadders-Algra M. Effects of long-chain polyunsaturated fatty acid supplementation of infant formula on cognition and behaviour at 9 years of age. Dev Med Child Neurol. 2012;54(12):1102-1108. doi:10.1111/j.1469-8749.2012.04444.x

707 Makrides M, Neumann MA, Simmer K, Gibson RA. A critical appraisal of the role of dietary long-chain polyunsaturated fatty acids on neural indices of term infants: a randomized, controlled trial. Pediatrics. 2000;105(1 Pt 1):32–38. doi:10.1542/peds.105.1.32

708 Makrides M, Gibson RA, McPhee AJ, et al. Effect of DHA supplementation during pregnancy on maternal depression and neurodevelopment of young children: a randomized controlled trial. JAMA. 2010;304(15):1675-1683. doi:10.1001/jama.2010.1507

709 Scott DT, Janowsky JS, Carroll RE, Taylor JA, Auestad N, Montalto MB. Formula supplementation with long-chain polyunsaturated fatty acids: are there developmental benefits?. Pediatrics. 1998;102(5):E59. doi:10.1542/peds.102.5.e59

710 de Groot RH, Adam J, Jolles J, Hornstra. Alpha-linolenic acid supplementation during human pregnancy does not effect cognitive functioning. Prostaglandins Leukot Essent Fatty Acids. 2004;70(1):41-47. doi:10.1016/j.plefa.2003.08.004

711 Lauritzen L, Jørgensen MH, Olsen SF, Straarup EM, Michaelsen KF. Maternal fish oil supplementation in lactation: effect on developmental outcome in breast-fed infants. Reprod Nutr Dev. 2005;45(5):535-547. doi:10.1051/rnd:2005044

712 Brantsæter AL, Birgisdottir BE, Meltzer HM, et al. Maternal seafood consumption and infant birth weight, length and head circumference in the Norwegian Mother and Child Cohort Study. Br J Nutr. 2012;107(3):436-444. doi:10.1017/S0007114511003047

713 Molloy CS, Stokes S, Makrides M, Collins CT, Anderson PJ, Doyle LW. Long-term effect of high-dose supplementation with DHA on visual function at school age in children born at <33 wk gestational age: results from a follow-up of a randomized controlled trial. Am J Clin Nutr. 2016;103(1):268-275. doi:10.3945/ajcn.115.114710

714 Harper KN, Hibbeln JR, Deckelbaum R, Quesenberry CP Jr, Schaefer CA, Brown AS. Maternal serum docosahexaenoic acid and schizophrenia spectrum disorders in adult offspring. Schizophr Res. 2011;128(1-3):30–36. doi:10.1016/j.schres.2011.01.009

715 Ramakrishnan U, Stinger A, DiGirolamoAM, Martorell R, Neufeld LM, Rivera JA, et al. (2015)Prenatal Docosahexaenoic Acid Supplementationand Offspring Development at 18 Months:Randomized Controlled Trial. PLoS ONE 10(8):e0120065. doi:10.1371/journal.pone.0120065

716 Mol Nutr Food Res. 2008 Dec;52(12):1478-85. doi: 10.1002/mnfr.200700451. Oxidation products of polyunsaturated fatty acids in infant formulas compared to human milk--a preliminary study. Michalski MC1, Calzada C, Makino A, Michaud S, Guichardant M.

717 Food Addit Contam. 2007 Nov;24(11):1209-18.
4-hydroxy-2-alkenals in polyunsaturated fatty acids-fortified infant formulas and other commercial food products.
Surh J1, Lee S, Kwon H.

718 Wainwright, P. E., Huang, Y.-S., Coscina, D. V., Lévesque, S., & McCutcheon, D. (1994). Brain and behavioral effects of dietary n-3 deficiency in mice: A three generational study. Developmental Psychobiology, 27(7), 467–487. https://doi.org/10.1002/dev.420270705

719 P.E. Wainwright, Y.-S. Huang, B. Bulman-Fleming, S. Lévesque, D. McCutcheon, The effects of dietary fatty acid composition combined with environmental enrichment on brain and behavior in mice, Behavioural Brain Research, Volume 60, Issue 2, 1994, Pages 125-136, ISSN 0166-4328, https://doi.org/10.1016/0166-4328(94)90139-2. (http://www.sciencedirect.com/science/article/pii/0166432894901392)

720 720 Carrié I, Guesnet P, Bourre JM, Francès H. Diets containing long-chain n-3 polyunsaturated fatty acids affect behaviour differently during development than ageing in mice. Br J Nutr. 2000;83(4):439-447

721 Saste MD, Carver JD, Stockard JE, Benford VJ, Chen LT, Phelps CP. Maternal diet fatty acid composition affects neurodevelopment in rat pups. J Nutr. 1998;128(4):740-743. doi:10.1093/jn/128.4.740

722 Church MW, Jen KL, Jackson DA, Adams BR, Hotra JW. Abnormal neurological responses in young adult offspring caused by excess omega-3 fatty acid (fish oil) consumption by the mother during pregnancy and lactation. Neurotoxicol Teratol. 2009;31(1):26-33. doi:10.1016/j.ntt.2008.09.001

723 Kehrer JP, Autor AP. Relationship between fatty acids and lipid peroxidation in lungs of neonates. Biol Neonate. 1978;34(1-2):61–67. doi:10.1159/000241106

724 Simmer K. Long-chain polyunsaturated fatty acid supplementation in infants born at term. Cochrane Database Syst Rev. 2001;(4):CD000376. doi:10.1002/14651858.CD000376

725 Auestad N, Halter R, Hall RT, et al. Growth and development in term infants fed long-chain polyunsaturated fatty acids: a double-masked, randomized, parallel, prospective, multivariate study. Pediatrics. 2001;108(2):372-381. doi:10.1542/peds.108.2.372

726 Grenyer BF, Crowe T, Meyer B, et al. Fish oil supplementation in the treatment of major depression: a randomised double-blind placebo-controlled trial. Prog Neuropsychopharmacol Biol Psychiatry. 2007;31(7):1393-1396. doi:10.1016/j.pnpbp.2007.06.004

727 Ghys A, Bakker E, Hornstra G, van den Hout M. Red blood cell and plasma phospholipid arachidonic and docosahexaenoic acid levels at birth and cognitive development at 4 years of age. Early Hum Dev. 2002;69(1-2):83-90. doi:10.1016/s0378-3782(02)00067-1

728 Birch, David & Birch, Eileen & Hoffman, Dennis & Uauy, Ricardo. (1992). Retinal Development in Very-Low-Birth-Weight Infants Fed Diets Differing in Omega-3 Fatty Acids. Investigative ophthalmology & visual science. 33. 2365-76

729 Robert E. Anderson, Maureen B. Maude, Lipids of ocular tissues: VIII. The effects of essential fatty acid deficiency on the phospholipids of the photoreceptor membranes of rat retina, Archives of Biochemistry and Biophysics, Volume 151, Issue 1, 1972, Pages 270-276, ISSN 0003-9861, https://doi.org/10.1016/0003-9861(72)90497-3. (http://www.sciencedirect.com/science/article/pii/0003986172904973)

730 Makrides M, Neumann MA, Byard RW, Simmer K, Gibson RA. Fatty acid composition of brain, retina, and erythrocytes in breast- and formula-fed infants. Am J Clin Nutr. 1994;60(2):189-194. doi:10.1093/ajcn/60.2.189

731 Tanito M, Brush RS, Elliott MH, Wicker LD, Henry KR, Anderson RE. High levels of retinal membrane docosahexaenoic acid increase susceptibility to stress-induced degeneration. J Lipid Res. 2009;50(5):807-819. doi:10.1194/jlr.M800170-JLR200

732 Li F, Marchette LD, Brush RS, et al. High levels of retinal docosahexaenoic acid do not protect photoreceptor degeneration in VPP transgenic mice. Mol Vis. 2010;16:1669-1679. Published 2010 Aug 18

733 Auestad N, Montalto MB, Hall RT, et al. Visual acuity, erythrocyte fatty acid composition, and growth in term infants fed formulas with long chain polyunsaturated fatty acids for one year. Ross Pediatric Lipid Study. Pediatr Res. 1997;41(1):1-10. doi:10.1203/00006450-199701000-00001

734 Goosey JD, Tuan WM, Garcia CA. A lipid peroxidative mechanism for posterior subcapsular cataract formation in the rabbit: a possible model for cataract formation in tapetoretinal diseases. Invest Ophthalmol Vis Sci. 1984;25(5):608-612

735 Borchman D, Stimmelmayr R, George JC. Whales, lifespan, phospholipids, and cataracts. J Lipid Res. 2017;58(12):2289-2298. doi:10.1194/jlr.M079368

736 Girao H, Mota C, Pereira P. Cholesterol may act as an antioxidant in lens membranes. Curr Eye Res. 1999;18(6):448-454. doi:10.1076/ceyr.18.6.448.5273

737 Girão H, Mota MC, Ramalho J, Pereira P. Cholesterol oxides accumulate in human cataracts. Exp Eye Res. 1998;66(5):645-652. doi:10.1006/exer.1998.0465

738 Ambaw YA, Chao C, Ji S, et al. Tear eicosanoids in healthy people and ocular surface disease. Sci Rep. 2018;8(1):11296. Published 2018 Jul 26. doi:10.1038/s41598-018-29568-3

739 BELL PG, O'NEILL JC. Optic atrophy in Hong Kong prisoners of war. Can Med Assoc J. 1947;56(5):475-481

740 SCHNITKER MA, MATTMAN PE, BLISS TL. A clinical study of malnutrition in Japanese prisoners of war. Ann Intern Med. 1951;35(1):69-96. doi:10.7326/0003-4819-35-1-69

741 Stevenson DS. Famine Oedema in Prisoners of War. Br Med J. 1944;1(4349):658-660. doi:10.1136/bmj.1.4349.658

742 Pradas I, Huynh K, Cabré R, Ayala V, Meikle PJ, Jové M and Pamplona R (2018) Lipidomics Reveals a Tissue-Specific Fingerprint. Front. Physiol. 9:1165. doi: 10.3389/fphys.2018.01165

743 THANNHAUSER SJ, BONCODDO NF, SCHMIDT G. Studies of acetal phospholipides of brain. I. Procedure of isolation of crystallized acetal phospholipide from brain. J Biol Chem. 1951;188(1):417-421

744 Skorve J, Hilvo M, Vihervaara T, et al. Fish oil and krill oil differentially modify the liver and brain lipidome when fed to mice. Lipids Health Dis. 2015;14:88. Published 2015 Aug 11. doi:10.1186/s12944-015-0086-2

745 Hurtado de Catalfo GE, de Alaniz MJ, Marra CA. Dietary lipids modify redox homeostasis and steroidogenic status in rat testis. Nutrition. 2008;24(7-8):717-726. doi:10.1016/j.nut.2008.03.008

746 Khan M, Singh J, Singh I. Plasmalogen deficiency in cerebral adrenoleukodystrophy and its modulation by lovastatin. J Neurochem. 2008;106(4):1766-1779. doi:10.1111/j.1471-4159.2008.05513.x

747 Reiss D, Beyer K, Engelmann B. Delayed oxidative degradation of polyunsaturated diacyl phospholipids in the presence of plasmalogen phospholipids in vitro. Biochem J. 1997;323 (Pt 3)(Pt 3):807-814. doi:10.1042/bj3230807

748 Rabetafika, Eric & Carreau, Jean-Paul. (1997). Peroxisomes and Essential Fatty Acid Deficiency.. Journal of Clinical Biochemistry and Nutrition. 23. 155-163. 10.3164/jcbn.23.155

749 Sztriha L, Al-Gazali LI, Wanders RJ, Ofman R, Nork M, Lestringant GG. Abnormal myelin formation in rhizomelic chondrodysplasia punctata type 2 (DHAPAT-deficiency). Dev Med Child Neurol. 2000;42(7):492-495. doi:10.1017/s0012162200000918

750 de Meijer VE, Kalish BT, Meisel JA, Le HD, Puder M. Dietary fish oil aggravates paracetamol-induced liver injury in mice. JPEN J Parenter Enteral Nutr. 2013;37(2):268-273. doi:10.1177/0148607112450735

751 Korkmaz H, Temel T, Bugdaci MS, Tekelioglu Y, Ozoran Y, Kapicioglu S. Effects of fish oil on cell proliferation and liver injury in an experimental model of acute hepatic injury induced by carbon tetrachloride. Bratisl Lek Listy. 2014;115(4):185-189. doi:10.4149/bll_2014_039

752 Paltauf F. Plasmalogen biosynthesis in a cell-free system. Enzymic desaturation of 1-O-alkyl (2-acyl) glycerophosphoryl ethanolamine. FEBS Lett. 1972;20(1):79-82. doi:10.1016/0014-5793(72)80021-8

753 Ruyter B, Lund JS, Thomassen MS, Christiansen EN. Studies of dihydroxyacetone phosphate acyltransferase in rat small intestine. Subcellular localization and effect of partially hydrogenated fish oil and clofibrate. Biochem J. 1992;282 (Pt 2)(Pt 2):565-570. doi:10.1042/bj2820565

754 Matheson, D. F., et al. "Changes in the Fatty Acyl Composition of Phospholipids in the Optic Tectum and Optic Nerve of

Temperature-Acclimated Goldfish." Physiological Zoology, vol. 53, no. 1, 1980, pp. 57–69. JSTOR, www.jstor.org/stable/30155775

755 Moukarzel S, Dyer RA, Keller BO, Elango R, Innis SM. Human Milk Plasmalogens Are Highly Enriched in Long-Chain PUFAs. J Nutr. 2016;146(11):2412-2417. doi:10.3945/jn.116.236802

756 Garcia C, Lutz NW, Confort-Gouny S, Cozzone PJ, Armand M, Bernard M. Phospholipid fingerprints of milk from different mammalians determined by 31P NMR: towards specific interest in human health. Food Chem. 2012;135(3):1777-1783. doi:10.1016/j.foodchem.2012.05.111

757 Sara Moukarzel, Roger A Dyer, Bernd O Keller, Rajavel Elango, Sheila M Innis, Human Milk Plasmalogens Are Highly Enriched in Long-Chain PUFAs, The Journal of Nutrition, Volume 146, Issue 11, November 2016, Pages 2412–2417, https://doi.org/10.3945/jn.116.236802

758 Karnati HK, Panigrahi MK, Li Y, Tweedie D, Greig NH. Adiponectin as a Potential Therapeutic Target for Prostate Cancer. Curr Pharm Des. 2017;23(28):4170-4179. doi:10.2174/1381612823666170208123553

759 Karnati HK, Panigrahi MK, Li Y, Tweedie D, Greig NH. Adiponectin as a Potential Therapeutic Target for Prostate Cancer. Curr Pharm Des. 2017;23(28):4170-4179. doi:10.2174/1381612823666170208123553

760 Barbosa MM, Melo AL, Damasceno NR. The benefits of ω-3 supplementation depend on adiponectin basal level and adiponectin increase after the supplementation: A randomized clinical trial. Nutrition. 2017;34:7-13. doi:10.1016/j.nut.2016.08.010

761 Page ST, Herbst KL, Amory JK, et al. Testosterone administration suppresses adiponectin levels in men. J Androl. 2005;26(1):85-92

762 Poehls J, Wassel CL, Harris TB, et al. Association of adiponectin with mortality in older adults: the Health, Aging, and Body Composition Study. Diabetologia. 2009;52(4):591-595. doi:10.1007/s00125-009-1261-7

763 Persson J, Folkersen L, Ekstrand J, et al. High plasma adiponectin concentration is associated with all-cause mortality in patients with carotid atherosclerosis. Atherosclerosis. 2012;225(2):491-496. doi:10.1016/j.atherosclerosis.2012.09.036

764 Lindberg S, Pedersen SH, Møgelvang R, et al. Usefulness of adiponectin as a predictor of all cause mortality in patients with ST-segment elevation myocardial infarction treated with primary percutaneous coronary intervention. Am J Cardiol. 2012;109(4):492-496. doi:10.1016/j.amjcard.2011.09.041

765 Wannamethee SG, Whincup PH, Lennon L, Sattar N. Circulating Adiponectin Levels and Mortality in Elderly Men With and Without Cardiovascular Disease and Heart Failure. Arch Intern Med. 2007;167(14):1510–1517. doi:10.1001/archinte.167.14.1510

766 Ortega Moreno L, Copetti M, Fontana A, et al. Evidence of a causal relationship between high serum adiponectin levels and increased cardiovascular mortality rate in patients with type 2 diabetes. Cardiovasc Diabetol. 2016;15:17. Published 2016 Jan 27. doi:10.1186/s12933-016-0339-z

767 Qiao L, Yoo Hs, Bosco C, et al. Adiponectin reduces thermogenesis by inhibiting brown adipose tissue activation in mice. Diabetologia. 2014;57(5):1027-1036. doi:10.1007/s00125-014-3180-5

768 Ealey KN, Kaludjerovic J, Archer MC, Ward WE. Adiponectin is a negative regulator of bone mineral and bone strength in growing mice. Exp Biol Med (Maywood). 2008;233(12):1546-1553. doi:10.3181/0806-RM-192

769 Lacasse JR, Leo J (2005) Serotonin and Depression: A Disconnect between the Advertisements and the Scientific Literature. PLoS Med 2(12): e392. https://doi.org/10.1371/journal.pmed.0020392

770 Patrick RP, Ames BN. Vitamin D and the omega-3 fatty acids control serotonin synthesis and action, part 2: relevance for ADHD, bipolar disorder, schizophrenia, and impulsive behavior. FASEB J. 2015;29(6):2207-2222. doi:10.1096/fj.14-268342

771 Nicoletti F, Raffaele R, Falsaperla A, Paci R. Circadian variation in 5-hydroxyindoleacetic acid levels in human cerebrospinal fluid. Eur Neurol. 1981;20(1):9-12. doi:10.1159/000115197

772 Sullivan GM, Oquendo MA, Huang YY, Mann JJ. Elevated cerebrospinal fluid 5-hydroxyindoleacetic acid levels in women with comorbid depression and panic disorder. Int J Neuropsychopharmacol. 2006;9(5):547-556. doi:10.1017/S1461145705006231

773 Bach H, Huang YY, Underwood MD, Dwork AJ, Mann JJ, Arango V. Elevated serotonin and 5-HIAA in the brainstem and lower serotonin turnover in the prefrontal cortex of suicides. Synapse. 2014;68(3):127-130. doi:10.1002/syn.21695

774 Sekiduka-Kumano T, Kawayama T, Ito K, et al. Positive association between the plasma levels of 5-hydroxyindoleacetic acid and the severity of depression in patients with chronic obstructive pulmonary disease. BMC Psychiatry. 2013;13:159. Published 2013 May 31. doi:10.1186/1471-244X-13-159

775 Coplan JD, Fulton SL, Reiner W, Jackowski A, Panthangi V, Perera TD, Gorman JM, Huang Y, Tang CY, Hof PR, Kaffman A, Dwork AJ, Mathew SJ, Kaufman J and Mann JJ (2014) Elevated cerebrospinal fluid 5-hydroxyindoleacetic acid in macaques following early life stress and inverse association with hippocampal volume: preliminary implications for serotonin-related function in mood and anxiety disorders. Front. Behav. Neurosci. 8:440. doi: 10.3389/fnbeh.2014.00440

776 Akkaya-Kalayci T, Kapusta ND, Waldhör T, Blüml V, Poustka L, Özlü-Erkilic Z. The association of monthly, diurnal and circadian variations with suicide attempts by young people. Child Adolesc Psychiatry Ment Health. 2017;11:35. Published 2017 Aug 1. doi:10.1186/s13034-017-0171-6

777 Perlis ML, Grandner MA, Brown GK, et al. Nocturnal Wakefulness as a Previously Unrecognized Risk Factor for Suicide. J Clin Psychiatry. 2016;77(6):e726-e733. doi:10.4088/JCP.15m10131

778 JOURNAL ARTICLE Some Neurophysiological Of Serotonin D. W. Woolley and E. Shaw The British Medical Journal Vol. 2, No. 4880 (Jul. 17, 1954), pp. 122-126

779 JOURNAL ARTICLE Some Neurophysiological Of Serotonin D. W. Woolley and E. Shaw The British Medical Journal Vol. 2, No. 4880 (Jul. 17, 1954), pp. 122-126

780 JOURNAL ARTICLE Some Neurophysiological Of Serotonin D. W. Woolley and E. Shaw The British Medical Journal Vol. 2, No. 4880 (Jul. 17, 1954), pp. 122-126

781 Mahler, D. J., & Humoller, F. L. (1968). The Influence of Serotonin on Oxidative Metabolism of Brain Mitochondria. Proceedings of the Society for Experimental Biology and Medicine, 127(4), 1074–1079. https://doi.org/10.3181/00379727-127-32874

782 Lin, M.T., Chow, C.F., Chern, Y.F. et al. Elevating serotonin levels in brain with 5-hydroxytryptophan produces hypothermia in rats. Pflugers Arch. 377, 245–249 (1978). https://doi.org/10.1007/BF00584279

783 Shestopalova, L.V., Vinogradova, M.S. & Dubinin, E.V. Seasonal dynamics of serotonin in the duodenum of hibernating animals. Bull Exp Biol Med 118, 1208–1210 (1994). https://doi.org/10.1007/BF02444627

784 Partington MW, Tu JB, Wong CY. Blood serotonin levels in severe mental retardation. Dev Med Child Neurol. 1973;15(5):616-627. doi:10.1111/j.1469-8749.1973.tb05172.x

785 Campbell M, Friedman E, Green WH, Collins PJ, Small AM, Breuer H. Blood serotonin in schizophrenic children. A preliminary study. Int Pharmacopsychiatry. 1975;10(4):213-221. doi:10.1159/000468197

786 Naffah-Mazzacoratti MG, Rosenberg R, Fernandes MJ, et al. Serum serotonin levels of normal and autistic children. Braz J Med Biol Res. 1993;26(3):309-317

787 Kuperman S, Beeghly J, Burns T, Tsai L. Association of serotonin concentration to behavior and IQ in autistic children. J Autism Dev Disord. 1987;17(1):133-140. doi:10.1007/BF01487265

788 Cook EH Jr, Leventhal BL, Freedman DX. Serotonin and measured intelligence. J Autism Dev Disord. 1988;18(4):553-559. doi:10.1007/BF02211873

789 Saxena J, Singh PN, Srivastava U, Siddiqui AQ. A study of thyroid hormones (t(3), t(4) & tsh) in patients of depression. Indian J Psychiatry. 2000;42(3):243-246

790 Skorve, Jon & Hilvo, Mika & Vihervaara, Terhi & Burri, Lena & Bohov, Pavol & Tillander, Veronika & Bjørndal, Bodil & Suoniemi, Matti & Laaksonen, Reijo & Ekroos, Kim & Berge, Rolf & Alexson, Stefan. (2015). Fish oil and krill oil differentially modify the liver and brain lipidome when fed to mice. Lipids in health and disease. 14. 88. 10.1186/s12944-015-0086-2

791 Bhattacharyya TK, Debnath PK. Role of 5-hydroxytryptamine in toxaemia of pregnancy. Indian J Physiol Pharmacol. 1995;39(1):86-88

792 Ghia, Jean-Eric & Li, Nan & Wang, Huaqing & Collins, Matthew & Deng, Yikang & El-Sharkawy, Rami & Francine, Côté & Mallet, Jacques & Khan, Waliul. (2009). Serotonin Has a Key Role in Pathogenesis of Experimental Colitis. Gastroenterology. 137. 1649-60. 10.1053/j.gastro.2009.08.041

793 Serotonin depletion eliminates sex differences with respect to context-conditioned immobility in rat. Robert Pettersson, Sven Melker Hagsäter, Elias Eriksson Psychopharmacology (Berl) 2016 Apr; 233(8): 1513–1521. Published online 2016 Feb 24. doi: 10.1007/s00213-016-4246-5

794 Angoa-Pérez M, Kane MJ, Briggs DI, et al. Mice genetically depleted of brain serotonin do not display a depression-like behavioral phenotype. ACS Chem Neurosci. 2014;5(10):908-919. doi:10.1021/cn500096g

795 Greenway, S.E., Pack, A.T. and Greenway, F.L. (1995), Treatment of Depression With Cyproheptadine. Pharmacotherapy: The Journal of Human Pharmacology and Drug Therapy, 15: 357-360. doi:10.1002/j.1875-9114.1995.tb04374.x

796 Halmi KA, Eckert E, LaDu TJ, Cohen J. Anorexia Nervosa: Treatment Efficacy of Cyproheptadine and Amitriptyline. Arch Gen Psychiatry. 1986;43(2):177–181. doi:10.1001/archpsyc.1986.01800020087011

797 Ruddell RG, Oakley F, Hussain Z, et al. A role for serotonin (5-HT) in hepatic stellate cell function and liver fibrosis. Am J Pathol. 2006;169(3):861-876. doi:10.2353/ajpath.2006.050767

798 R.E Grahn, M.J Will, S.E Hammack, S Maswood, M.B McQueen, L.R Watkins, S.F Maier, Activation of serotonin-immunoreactive cells in the dorsal raphe nucleus in rats exposed to an uncontrollable stressor, Brain Research, Volume 826, Issue 1, 1999, Pages 35-43, ISSN 0006-8993, https://doi.org/10.1016/S0006-8993(99)01208-1

799 Antibodies to serotonin attenuate closed head injury induced blood brain barrier disruption and brain pathology. H. S. Sharma, R. Patnaik, S. Patnaik, S. Mohanty, A. Sharma, P. Vannemreddy Ann N Y Acad Sci. 2007 Dec; 1122: 295–312. doi: 10.1196/annals.1403.022

800 Rybaczyk, Leszek & Bashaw, Meredith & Pathak, Dorothy & Moody, Scott & Gilders, Roger & Holzschu, Donald. (2005). An overlooked connection: Serotonergic mediation of estrogen-related physiology and pathology. BMC women's health. 5. 12. 10.1186/1472-6874-5-12

801 AU - Anne Lorraine Smazal AU - Kevin Lee Schalinske TI - Oral Administration of Retinoic Acid Lowers Brain Serotonin Concentration in Rats PT - Journal Article DP - 2013 TA - The FASEB Journal PG - 635.6-635.6 VI - 27 IP - 1_supplement AID - 10.1096/fasebj.27.1_supplement.635.6 [doi] 4099 - https://www.fasebj.org/doi/abs/10.1096/fasebj.27.1_supplement.635.6 4100 - https://www.fasebj.org/doi/full/10.1096/fasebj.27.1_supplement.635.6 SO - The FASEB Journal April 2013 27(1_supplement):635.6 AB

802 Hidehiko Yokogoshi, Kimiko Oishi & Misako Okitsu (1993) Accumulation of Brain Tryptophan in Rats after Administering Various Fats or Fatty Acids, Bioscience, Biotechnology, and Biochemistry, 57:2, 181-184, DOI: 10.1271/bbb.57.181

803 Aviram M, Cogan U, Mokady S. Excessive dietary tryptophan enhances plasma lipid peroxidation in rats. Atherosclerosis. 1991;88(1):29-34. doi:10.1016/0021-9150(91)90254-z

804 McNamara RK, Able J, Liu Y, et al. Omega-3 fatty acid deficiency during perinatal development increases serotonin turnover in the prefrontal cortex and decreases midbrain tryptophan hydroxylase-2 expression in

adult female rats: dissociation from estrogenic effects. J Psychiatr Res. 2009;43(6):656-663. doi:10.1016/j.jpsychires.2008.09.011

805 Sidransky, H. Dietary tryptophan and aging. Amino Acids 13, 91–103 (1997). https://doi.org/10.1007/BF01373208

806 GROWTH ON DIETS POOR IN TRUE FATS. BY THOMAS B. OSBORNE AND LAFAYETTE B. MENDEL. (From the Laboratory of the Connecticut Agricultural Experiment Station and the Shefield Laboratory of Physiological Chemistry, Yale University, New Haven.) (Received for publication, October 21, 1920..

807 Hindhede, M.: Skand. Arch. f. Physiol. 30:78, 1913;Hindhede,M.:Skand. Arch.f.Physiol.30:78,1913;publishedinGermanin1919. Researchwasbegun,Aug.25,1916.ByApril4,1917,"after nine months 'experience with a fat free diet, we were convinced that adults could live without fats, provided they were given greens

808 William Redman Brown, Arild Edsten Hansen, George Oswald Burr, Irvine McQuarrie, Effects of Prolonged Use of Extremely Low-Fat Diet on an Adult Human Subject, The Journal of Nutrition, Volume 16, Issue 6, December 1938, Pages 511–524, https://doi.org/10.1093/jn/16.6.511

809 McAmis, Ava & Anderson, William & Mendel, Lafayette. (1929). Growth of rats on "fat-Free" diets. Journal of Biological Chemistry. 82. 247-262

810 810 Hindhede,M.,Molkerei-Ztg.,1918,xxviii,152;abstractedinChem. Zentr.,1918,ii,745;Skand.Arch.Physiol.,1920,xxxix,78

811 A New Deficiency Disease Produced by the Rigid Exclusion of Fat from the Diet (Burr, G. O., and Burr, M. M. (1929) J. Biol. Chem. 82, 345–367)

812 Essential Fatty Acids: The Work of George and Mildred Burr. The Journal of Biological Chemistry. 2012;287(42):35439-35441. doi:10.1074/jbc. O112.000005

813 A. Skalli, J.H. Robin, N. Le Bayon, H. Le Delliou, J. Person-Le Ruyet, Impact of essential fatty acid deficiency and temperature on tissues' fatty acid composition of European sea bass (Dicentrarchus labrax), Aquaculture, Volume 255, Issues 1–4, 2006, Pages 223-232, ISSN 0044-8486, https:// doi.org/10.1016/j.aquaculture.2005.12.006.http://www.sciencedirect.com/ science/article/pii/S004484860500760X

814 Hume EM, Smith HH. The relation of a fat-free diet to the scaly tail condition in rats described by Burr and Burr. Biochem J. 1931;25(1):300– 306. doi:10.1042/bj0250300

815 H. Schneider, H. Steenbock, and Blanche R. Platz ESSENTIAL FATTY ACIDS, VITAMIN B6, AND OTHER FACTORS IN THE CURE OF RAT ACRODYNIA J. Biol. Chem. 1940 132: 539

816 F. W. Quackenbush, H. Steenbock, F. A. Kummerow, B. R. Platz, Linoleic Acid, Pyridoxine and Pantothenic Acid in Rat Dermatitis, The Journal of Nutrition, Volume 24, Issue 3, September 1942, Pages 225–234, https://doi.org/10.1093/jn/24.3.225

817 Birch T.W. The Relation Between Vitamin B6 and Unsaturated Fatty Acid Factor. J. Biol. Chem. 1938; 124: 775

818 TANGE, Ume. (2011). Studies on Vitamin B2 Complex. VI Rat-acrodynia and Fatty Acids. Bulletin of the Agricultural Chemical Society of Japan. 21. 10.1271/bbb1924.16.21

819 Zehaluk CM, Walker BL. Effect of pyridoxine on red cell fatty acid composition in mature rats fed an essential fatty acid-deficient diet. J Nutr. 1973;103(11):1548–1553. doi:10.1093/jn/103.11.1548

820 Kim, Dong. (1961). Experimental Production of Arteriosclerosis in Rhesus Monkeys by Deficiency of Pyridoxine Hydrochloride (Vitamin B-6) and Essential Fatty Acids. Yonsei Medical Journal. 2. 42. 10.3349/ymj.1961.2.1.42

821 Bettger WJ, Reeves PG, Moscatelli EA, Reynolds G, O'Dell BL. Interaction of zinc and essential fatty acids in the rat. J Nutr. 1979;109(3):480–488. doi:10.1093/jn/109.3.480

822 Wauben IP, Xing HC, Wainwright PE. Neonatal dietary zinc deficiency in artificially reared rat pups retards behavioral development and interacts with essential fatty acid deficiency to alter liver and brain fatty acid composition. J Nutr. 1999;129(10):1773–1781. doi:10.1093/jn/129.10.1773

823 Roth HP, Kirchgessner M. Einfluss des Diätfettes auf die Hämolyseresistenz der Erythrozytenmembran bei alimentärem Zn- bzw. Ca-Mangel bei der Ratte [The effect of dietary fats on the hemolysis resistance of the erythrocyte membrane during alimentary zinc and calcium deficiency in rats]. Z Ernahrungswiss. 1991;30(2):98–108. doi:10.1007/bf01610065

824 Biervliet, Stephanie. (2008). Zinc and essential fatty acid status and supplementation in cystic fibrosis patients. Journal du Pédiatre Belge. 10. 64-66

825 Parsons HG, O'Loughlin EV, Forbes D, Cooper D, Gall DG. Supplemental calories improve essential fatty acid deficiency in cystic fibrosis patients. Pediatr Res. 1988;24(3):353–356. doi:10.1203/00006450-198809000-00016

826 Bailey, B.. (2011). Fish Oils.: IX. Certain Fish Oils as Sources of Nutritionally Essential Fatty Acids.. Journal of the Fisheries Research Board of Canada. 109-112. 10.1139/f42-013

827 Bazinet RP, Douglas H, Cunnane SC. Whole-body utilization of n-3 PUFA in n-6 PUFA-deficient rats. Lipids. 2003;38(2):187–189. doi:10.1007/s11745-003-1050-8

828 1964. SMITH JA, DELUCA HF. STRUCTURAL CHANGES IN ISOLATED LIVER MITOCHONDRIA OF RATS DURING ESSENTIAL FATTY ACID DEFICIENCY. J Cell Biol. 1964;21(1):15–26. doi:10.1083/jcb.21.1.15

829 Drummond JC, Coward KH. Researches on the Fat-soluble Accessory Substance. III: Technique for carrying out Feeding Tests for Vitamin A (Fat-soluble A). Biochem J. 1920;14(5):661–664. doi:10.1042/bj0140661

830 Bibel DJ, Miller SJ, Brown BE, et al. Antimicrobial activity of stratum corneum lipids from normal and essential fatty acid-deficient mice. J Invest Dermatol. 1989;92(4):632–638. doi:10.1111/1523-1747.ep12712202

831 LIPIDS AND THYROID HORMONES FREDERIC L. HOCH, Departments of Internal Medicine and Biological Chemistry, The University of Michigan Medical School, Ann Arbor, Michigan 48109, U.S.A.

832 Forrest GL, Futterman S. Age-related changes in the retinal capillaries and the fatty acid composition of retinal tissue of normal and essential fatty acid-deficient rats. Invest Ophthalmol. 1972;11(9):760–764

833 Palsdottir V, Wickman A, Andersson N, et al. Postnatal deficiency of essential fatty acids in mice results in resistance to diet-induced obesity and low plasma insulin during adulthood. Prostaglandins Leukot Essent Fatty Acids. 2011;84(3-4):85–92. doi:10.1016/j.plefa.2010.11.002

834 Palsdottir V, Olsson B, Borén J, Strandvik B, Gabrielsson BG. Postnatal essential fatty acid deficiency in mice affects lipoproteins, hepatic lipids, fatty acids and mRNA expression. Prostaglandins Leukot Essent Fatty Acids. 2011;85(3-4):179–188. doi:10.1016/j.plefa.2011.05.002

835 Palsdottir V, Månsson JE, Blomqvist M, Egecioglu E, Olsson B. Long-term effects of perinatal essential fatty acid deficiency on anxiety-related behavior in mice. Behav Neurosci. 2012;126(2):361–369. doi:10.1037/a0027161

836 Ling PR, Malkan A, Le HD, Puder M, Bistrian BR. Arachidonic acid and docosahexaenoic acid supplemented to an essential fatty acid-deficient diet alters the response to endotoxin in rats. Metabolism. 2012;61(3):395–406. doi:10.1016/j.metabol.2011.07.017

837 Benhamou PY, Mullen Y, Clare-Salzler M, et al. Essential fatty acid deficiency prevents autoimmune diabetes in nonobese diabetic mice through a positive impact on antigen-presenting cells and Th2 lymphocytes. Pancreas. 1995;11(1):26-37. doi:10.1097/00006676-199507000-00003

838 Morganroth ML, Schoeneich SO, Till GO, Pickett W, Ward PA. Lung injury caused by cobra venom factor is reduced in rats raised on an essential fatty acid-deficient diet. Am J Physiol. 1989;257(4 Pt 2):H1192-H1199. doi:10.1152/ajpheart.1989.257.4.H1192

839 Ball HA, Cook JA, Spicer KM, Wise WC, Halushka PV. Essential fatty acid-deficient rats are resistant to oleic acid-induced pulmonary injury. J Appl Physiol (1985). 1989;67(2):811-816. doi:10.1152/jappl.1989.67.2.811

840 Wright JR Jr, Fraser RB, Kapoor S, Cook HW. Essential fatty acid deficiency prevents multiple low-dose streptozotocin-induced diabetes in naive and cyclosporin-treated low-responder murine strains. Acta Diabetol. 1995;32(2):125-130. doi:10.1007/bf00569571

841 Rovin BH, Lefkowith JB, Schreiner GF. Mechanisms underlying the anti-inflammatory effects of essential fatty acid deficiency in experimental glomerulonephritis. Inhibited release of a monocyte chemoattractant by glomeruli. J Immunol. 1990;145(4):1238-1245

842 Hurd ER, Gilliam JN. Beneficial effect of an essential fatty acid deficient diet in NZB/NZW F1 mice. J Invest Dermatol. 1981;77(5):381-384. doi:10.1111/1523-1747.ep12494224

843 Penturf ME, McGlone JJ, Griswold JA. Modulation of immune response in thermal injury by essential fatty acid-deficient diet. J Burn Care Rehabil. 1996;17(5):465-464

844 Mascolo N, Izzo AA, Autore G, Maiello FM, Di Carlo G, Capasso F. Acetic acid-induced colitis in normal and essential fatty acid deficient rats. J Pharmacol Exp Ther. 1995;272(1):469-475

845 Hargrave KM, Azain MJ, Miner JL. Dietary coconut oil increases conjugated linoleic acid-induced body fat loss in mice independent of essential fatty acid deficiency. Biochim Biophys Acta. 2005;1737(1):52-60. doi:10.1016/j.bbalip.2005.08.016

846 Porras-Reyes BH, Schreiner GF, Lefkowith JB, Mustoe TA. Essential fatty acids are not required for wound healing. Prostaglandins Leukot Essent Fatty Acids. 1992;45(4):293-298. doi:10.1016/0952-3278(92)90086-x

847 Albina JE, Gladden P, Walsh WR. Detrimental effects of an omega-3 fatty acid-enriched diet on wound healing. JPEN J Parenter Enteral Nutr. 1993;17(6):519–521. doi:10.1177/0148607193017006519

848 Smith SS, Neuringer M, Ojeda SR. Essential fatty acid deficiency delays the onset of puberty in the female rat. Endocrinology. 1989;125(3):1650–1659. doi:10.1210/endo-125-3-1650

849 Ahluwalia B, Shima S, Pincus G. In vitro synthesis of androgens by testicular tissue of rat deficient in essential fatty acids. J Reprod Fertil. 1968;17(2):263–273. doi:10.1530/jrf.0.0170263

850 B. AHLUWALIA, S. SHIMA, D. ALLMANN, In Vivo Biosynthesis of Testosterone in the Testes of the Essential Fatty Acid-Deficient Rat, Endocrinology, Volume 88, Issue 1, 1 January 1971, Pages 106–114, https://doi.org/10.1210/endo-88-1-106

851 Petrie JR, Shrestha P, Zhou XR, et al. Metabolic engineering plant seeds with fish oil-like levels of DHA. PLoS One. 2012;7(11):e49165. doi:10.1371/journal.pone.0049165

852 Salem N Jr, Eggersdorfer M. Is the world supply of omega-3 fatty acids adequate for optimal human nutrition?. Curr Opin Clin Nutr Metab Care. 2015;18(2):147–154. doi:10.1097/MCO.0000000000000145

853 Hu, Xingzhong and Chen, Dong and Wu, Lianpeng and He, Guiqing and Ye, Wei, Low Serum Cholesterol Level Among Patients with COVID-19 Infection in Wenzhou, China (February 21, 2020). Available at SSRN: https://ssrn.com/abstract=3544826 or http://dx.doi.org/10.2139/ssrn.3544826

854 BMJ 2020;368:m1182

855 Zheng, M., Gao, Y., Wang, G. et al. Functional exhaustion of antiviral lymphocytes in COVID-19 patients. Cell Mol Immunol 17, 533–535 (2020)

856 Xia, Sheng & Li, Xiaoping & Cheng, Lu & Han, Mutian & Zhang, Miaomiao & Liu, Xia & Xu, Hua-Xi & Zhang, Minghui & Shao, Qixiang & Qi, Ling. (2014). Chronic intake of high fish oil diet induces myeloid-derived suppressor cells to promote tumor growth. Cancer immunology, immunotherapy : CII. 63. 10.1007/s00262-014-1546-7

857 Schwerbrock NM, Karlsson EA, Shi Q, Sheridan PA, Beck MA. Fish oil-fed mice have impaired resistance to influenza infection. The Journal of Nutrition. 2009 Aug;139(8):1588-1594. DOI: 10.3945/jn.109.108027

858 Shahabi nezhad, F.; Mosaddeghi, P.; Negahdaripour, M.; Dehghani, Z.; Farahmandnejad, M.; Moghadami, M.; Nezafat, N.; Masoompour, S.M. Therapeutic Approaches for COVID-19 Based on the Dynamics of

Interferon-mediated Immune Responses. Preprints 2020, 2020030206 (doi: 10.20944/preprints202003.0206.v1)

859 Paul M. Byleveld, Gerald T. Pang, Robert L. Clancy, David C. K. Roberts, Fish Oil Feeding Delays Influenza Virus Clearance and Impairs Production of Interferon-γ and Virus-Specific Immunoglobulin A in the Lungs of Mice, The Journal of Nutrition, Volume 129, Issue 2, February 1999, Pages 328–335, https://doi.org/10.1093/jn/129.2.328

860 El-Kurdi B, Khatua B, Rood C, et al. MORTALITY FROM COVID-19 INCREASES WITH UNSATURATED FAT, AND MAY BE REDUCED BY EARLY CALCIUM AND ALBUMIN SUPPLEMENTATION [published online ahead of print, 2020 May 27]. *Gastroenterology*. 2020;S0016-5085(20)34727-2. doi:10.1053/j.gastro.2020.05.057